A PEARSON AUSTRALIA CUSTOM BOOK

ACADEMIC SKILLS FOR NURSING AND MIDWIFERY STUDENTS

This custom book is compiled from:

THE LITTLE PENGUIN HANDBOOK
2ND EDITION
FAIGLEY

WRITING FOR THE SOCIAL SCIENCES
RAGUSA

UNIVERSITY OF SOUTH AUSTRALIA

Pearson Australia
Unit 4, Level 3
14 Aquatic Drive
Frenchs Forest, Sydney NSW 2086
Ph: 02 9454 2200
www.pearson.com.au

Managing Editor: Jill Gillies
Consultant: Claire Sadler
Project Manager: Aida Reyes Cruz
Production Controller: Caroline Stewart

ISBN: 978 1 4860 1551 1

Printed and bound in Australia by The SOS Print + Media Group

Acknowledgements

This compilation has contributions from Dr. Maria Fedoruk. A special thank you should be also given to Pearson Education Consultant, Hanna Benson, for her involvement in the planning of this custom book edition.

Table of contents

1 Beginning university studies: Introduction

This book/primer on academic writing is a joint venture between the University of South Australia's School of Nursing & Midwifery, (SON&M) Learning and Teaching Unit (LTU) and Pearson Australia. This book has been adapted for local students from 'The Little Penguin Handbook by Lester Faigley and published in 2013.

The book has been developed to support students studying and writing at university for the first time and for students returning to study. This book will also be useful for international students to navigate the complexities of academic writing in Australian universities.

2 Writing as communication

Writing is a form of communication. Whether you are writing an essay for a nursing course; writing a report or preparing a presentation for your class you are engaging in the complex process of communication. The process of communication has three (3) main elements:

The writer/speaker

The audience

The subject

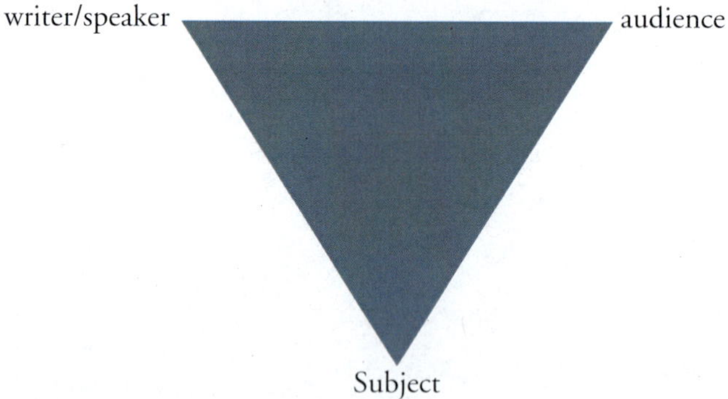

These three elements are necessary for communication to occur. As a speaker you make adjustments to your communication according to your audience. As a writer you are writing for a reader on a specific topic. Therefore, it is important that you understand your assessment topic and what you are being asked to do. Use the templates provided- for example: templates for care plans; report writing

3 Reflection

Reflect on how you communicate with family, friends, co-workers. Are there any differences?

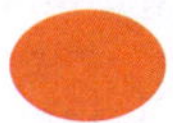

Think about your audience

As a student you write primarily for your lecturer and classmates. In the workplace or on clinical placement you may not know who will be reading your notes and reports.

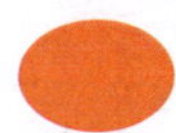

Reflection

Reflect on your professional writing – in the classroom; assignments; work-places/clinical placements- who is your audience? Will your writing style change according to your audience?

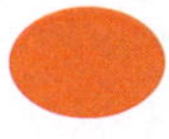

Learning & Teaching Unit – University of South Australia

http://resource.unisa.edu.au/course/view.php?id=3633&topic=7

This link will take you to the Learning & Teaching Unit's resources on academic writing. The resources are comprehensive and cover the principles of writing your assignments and other forms of written communication

http://resource.unisa.edu.au/course/view.php?id=3633&topic=4

This link will take you to the Learning & Teaching Unit's resources on specific types of assignments like essays, journals, reports and eportfolio items.

4 Reading

Reading is the important first step prior to writing an essay or assignment. The first thing you have to read and understand is the assessment task. What are you being asked to do? At UniSA you are expected to read critically and the following link will take you to a section on the LTU web site that discusses critical reading:
http://resource.unisa.edu.au/mod/book/view.php?id=4245&chapterid=1385

Faigley (2013) presents a series of questions for the critical reader to ask when reading articles, books, journals in preparation for writing an assignment:

- Who wrote this material?
- Where did it first appear? Books, newspapers; magazine or online? Is it a credible source? While GOOGLE and Wikipedia will give you ready access to information this may not always be credible or accurate. A hint here: It is better to use GOOGLE Scholar available via the university's web site @ http://www.library.unisa.edu.au/Default.aspx for your first attempt at looking for references for your assignment. GOOGLE Scholar provides refereed journals and books. The library enables access to data bases that will provide you with current reference material.
- What is the topic or issue? When gathering reference material it is easy to get side-tracked with other interesting pieces of information that you come across. Remember good assignment writing is focused on the topic.
- Does the writer have strong or not so strong opinions on the topic?
- What else has been written on the topic? How recent is this information? A rule of thumb here: use references that are no more than 5 years old unless they are the seminal works in a particular field such as theories of nursing, management, child development, mental health.
- Why was it written? Did it address a gap in knowledge?

Dealing with Difficult Readings

From time to time you will be set readings that are difficult. Difficulties may be because of length; language used by authors or it may be that the subject matter is unfamiliar to you. Strategies to deal with difficult readings include:

- skim read to get an overview of a reading
- preview layout and content (abstracts in journal articles do this)
- read the most important sections first
- you should be able to see the connection between the introduction and the conclusion
- scan for specific information
- make notes/summarise key points- either in the margins of journal articles (if reading on line you can do this using the review function in Word) or in note books. This helps you retain information

Even though you do not understand every word, see if you can get the main point(s) the author is making

- focus on key sections—introduction, conclusion, topic sentences
- if you are unfamiliar with specialised words to do with the topic, make a list of frequently-occurring words and try to find their meaning elsewhere (e.g. in a subject dictionary)
- if the problem words are not specialist words but just unfamiliar language, substitute words that would make sense
- compile a list of questions to find the answers elsewhere: other students, lecturers; a simpler text on the same topic.

5 Critical thinking and reasoning

You will have been introduced to critical thinking and reasoning in the first year of the program. Those students who have entered the program in second year may not yet have been introduced to critical thinking and analysis but will find this embedded in all the courses in the undergraduate nursing program.

Critical thinking is inherent in the Inquiry Based Learning Model that underpins the undergraduate curriculum in the SON&M. Critical thinking encourages the asking of questions about events: situations- for example why something has occurred.

Critical thinking enables you to reflect, connect, question, investigate, construct and express new knowledge. You will use critical thinking when analysing case studies for assessment. When reading critically ask the following questions:

- Who is the author?
- Does the author have expertise in this area?
- Where did this first appear? A refereed journal; a book chapter; the media (print & electronic)
- What is this about? What is the main focus of this piece of work?
- Does the writer(s) have an opinion on the issue and how well is this expressed?
- Is there any other material about this topic or issue?
- Why was this written? Was it in response to a media report? A coronial inquiry? Or a government report?

In this stage of your program your clinical placement experiences will also require you to think critically as you read documentation related to patient care. This documentation can be patient notes; medication orders etc.

6 Smart thinking

Allen (2012 pp1–2) calls critical thinking smart thinking. Smart thinking is:

- Being able to work out and express your ideas
- Plan your communication of ideas so that they can be clearly understood
- Check to see if you have covered the key areas of your topic
- Establish a framework or structure in which your basic facts and evidence make sense
- Present ideas by linking them together to convince your readers of your conclusion

Smart thinking is thinking with a purpose and all thinking is underpinned by reasoning. Reasoning enables you to understand and make sense of your world. Reasoning is something all people do but university studies help you develop your reasoning capabilities because you learn to make connections between different ideas and concepts.

7 Dealing with loss of concentration

Reading can be tiring – especially if the material is new to you and difficult to understand. You need to manage your time to read effectively which doesn't mean you have to spend hours at a time with your head in a book or journal articles. If you find you are losing concentration – take a break. Use the following strategies to help you understand what works for you when reading:

- work out how long you can sit and concentrate for at one time (30–50 minutes is average)
- if you are reading but nothing is going in – take a break
- take regular breaks away from the space you are reading in
- go for a walk to get some fresh air

8 Summarising

Make sure you understand exactly what the focus of the writer is. Underline/circle any words you do not understand and look them up or ask your lecturer. Summarise the main points by asking these questions:

- What is the writer's main claim or question?
- What are the key ideas/concepts?
- Do you agree with the author's claims?
- Use the strategies listed above to manage difficult readings

9 Elements of good writing

Elements of good writing include:

- Having a good vocabulary
- A discipline specific vocabulary
- Knowing the rules of grammar and punctuation
- Cultural nuances of English language
- Knowing how to construct an effective paragraph

Good writing is a form of communication. Therefore it makes sense to communicate effectively with your intended audience: lecturers; colleagues; communities of practice.

Good writing is evident when the vocabulary used suits the subject; words are not overused; text language/jargon are not used.

10 The writing process

All good writing begins with an idea of what is required and then this idea is made into an outline. The outline is a plan that shows how you are going to arrange the different sections of your written assignment. Once you have noted the main headings usually Introduction; main discussion & finally a conclusion. Under these three main headings begin to add the main points for each section and so gradually build up your assignment.

It is also a good idea to begin organising your references at this point. There is usually no set number of references to be used. The number of references used is up to you but one reference is not enough and 30 references for a 1,000 word assessment piece is too much. References support your emerging thesis/argument on a certain topic and are not central to your work. Write your references down and save in a safe place so that when you are ready for references you just need to go to your saved list. The library provides information on how to manage references.

Hint: references should be current no older than 5 years unless they are seminal works in a particular area for example: a particular theory that has not been disproved.

Once all your ideas are written down you should begin organising how you will present your ideas.

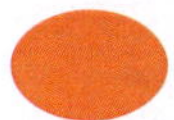

Introduction

The introduction should capture your reader's interest because it introduces your topic. The first sentence of the introduction should focus the reader's attention on the subject being discussed by you. The introduction should not be too long and should flow into the main discussion.

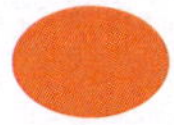

Main discussion

Each paragraph and sentence in this section should showcase your knowledge of the topic. Your emerging discussion should be supported with references. From reading the Harvard referencing guide discussed previously you will know how to reference correctly. The references you use support your point of view and not the other way around. A series of references punctuated by a brief sentence from you is not acceptable. The discussion should reflect your ideas and opinions.

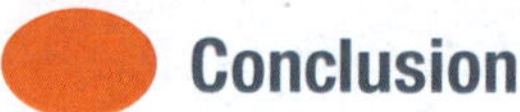

Conclusion

The conclusion summarises the content of the paper. New material should not be introduced in the conclusion.

11 Understanding Grammar

Good writing requires an understanding of how the effective use of grammar enhances the quality of your written work. The use of text language in academic writing is not appropriate.

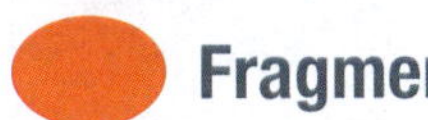

Fragments

Fragments are incomplete sentences. They are punctuated to look like sentences, but they lack a key element—often a subject or a verb—or else they are subordinate clauses or phrases. Consider this example of a full sentence followed by a fragment:

> The university's enrolment rose unexpectedly during the second semester. **Because the percentage of students who accepted offers of admission was much higher than in previous years and fewer students than usual dropped out or transferred.**

When a sentence starts with *because*, we expect to find a main clause later. Instead, the *because* clause refers back to the previous sentence. The writer no doubt knew that the fragment gave the reasons why enrolment rose, but a reader must stop to determine the connection.

In formal writing you should avoid fragments. Readers expect words punctuated as a sentence to be a complete sentence. They expect writers to complete their thoughts rather than force readers to guess the missing element.

Basic strategies for turning fragments into sentences

Incorporate the fragment into an adjoining sentence.

In many cases you can incorporate the fragment into an adjoining sentence.

> *game, playing*
> I was hooked on the ~~game. Playing~~ day and night.

Add the missing element.

If you cannot incorporate a fragment into another sentence, add the missing element.

> *investors should think*
>
> When aiming for the highest returns, ~~and also thinking~~ about the possible losses.

COMMON ERRORS

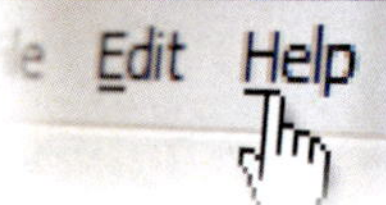

Recognising fragments

If you can spot fragments, you can fix them. Grammar checkers can find some of them, but they miss many fragments and may identify other sentences wrongly as fragments. Ask these questions when you are checking for sentence fragments.

- **Does the sentence have a subject?** Except for commands, sentences need subjects:

  Jane spent every cent of credit she had available. **And then applied for more cards.**

- **Does the sentence have a complete verb?** Sentences require complete verbs. Verbs that end in *-ing* must have an auxiliary verb to be complete.

  Robert keeps changing courses. **He trying to figure out what he really wants to do after university.**

- **If the sentence begins with a subordinate clause, is there a main clause in the same sentence?**

  Even though it is cheaper to watch a DVD than visit a movie theatre, it is the total experience that moviegoers enjoy. **Which is one reason people continue to go to the movies.**

Remember:

1. A sentence must have a subject and a complete verb.

2. A subordinate clause cannot stand alone as a sentence.

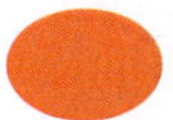

Run-on Sentences

While fragments are incomplete sentences, run-ons jam together two or more sentences, failing to separate them with appropriate punctuation.

Fixing run-on sentences

Take three steps to fix run-on sentences: (1) identify the problem, (2) determine where the run-on sentence needs to be divided, and (3) choose the punctuation that best indicates the relationship between the main clauses.

COMMON ERRORS

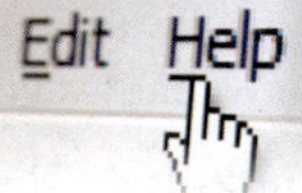

Recognising run-on sentences

When you read this sentence, you realise something is wrong.

> **I don't recall what kind of printer it was all I remember is that it could sort, staple and print a packet at the same time.**

The problem is that two main clauses aren't separated by punctuation. The reader must look carefully to determine where one main clause stops and the next one begins.

> I don't recall what kind of printer it was | all I remember is that it could sort, staple and print a packet at the same time.

A full stop should be placed after *was*, and the next sentence should begin with a capital letter:

> I don't recall what kind of printer it was. All I remember is that it could sort, staple and print a packet at the same time.

Run-on sentences are major errors.

Remember: Two main clauses must be separated by correct punctuation.

1. Identify the problem.

When you read your writing aloud, run-on sentences will often trip you up, just as they confuse readers. If you find two main clauses with no punctuation separating them, you have a run-on sentence. You can also search for subject and verb pairs to check for run-ons.

SUBJ VERB

Internet businesses are not bound to specific locations or old ways of running a business they are more flexible in allowing employees to telecommute and to determine the hours they work.

S V

2. Determine where the run-on sentence needs to be divided.

Internet businesses are not bound to specific locations or old ways of running a business | they are more flexible in allowing employees to telecommute and to determine the hours they work.

3. Determine the relationship between the main clauses.

You will revise a run-on more effectively if you first determine the relationship between the main clauses and understand the effect or point you are trying to make. There are several punctuation strategies for fixing run-ons.

- **Insert a full stop**. This is the simplest way to fix a run-on sentence.

  Internet businesses are not bound to specific locations or old ways of running a business. They are more flexible in allowing employees to telecommute and to determine the hours they work.

  However, if you want to indicate more clearly a closer relationship between the two main clauses, you may want to choose one of the following strategies.

- **Insert a semicolon (and possibly a transitional word specifying the relationship between the two main clauses).**

  Internet businesses are not bound to specific locations or old ways of running a business; therefore, they are more flexible in allowing employees to telecommute and to determine the hours they work.

- **Insert a comma and a coordinating conjunction (*and*, *but*, *or*, *nor*, *for*, *so*, *yet*).**

  Internet businesses are not bound to specific locations or old ways of running a business, so they are more flexible in allowing employees to telecommute and to determine the hours they work.

- **Make one of the clauses subordinate.**

  Because Internet businesses are not bound to specific locations or old ways of running a business, they are more flexible in allowing employees to telecommute and to determine the hours they work.

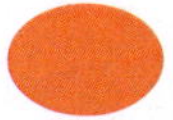

Comma Splices

Comma splices occur when two or more sentences are incorrectly joined by a comma: A comma links two clauses that could stand on their own. In this example, the comma following 'classes' should be a full stop.

> **Most of us were taking the same classes, if someone had a question, we would all help out.**

Such sentences include a punctuation mark—a comma—separating two main clauses. However, a comma isn't a strong enough punctuation mark to separate two main clauses.

Fixing comma splices

You have several options for fixing comma splices. Select the one that best fits where the sentence is located and the effect you are trying to achieve.

1. Change the comma to a full stop.

Most comma splices can be fixed by changing the comma to a full stop.

> It didn't matter that I worked in a windowless room for 40 hours a ~~week, on~~ *week. On* the Web I was exploring and learning more about distant people and places than I ever had before.

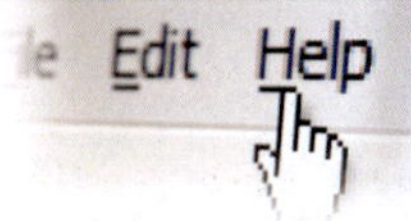

COMMON ERRORS

Recognising comma splices

When you edit your writing, look carefully at sentences that contain commas. Does the sentence contain two main clauses? If so, are the main clauses joined by a comma and coordinating conjunction (*and, but, for, or, not, so, yet*)?

COMMON ERRORS

Incorrect The **concept** of 'nature' **depends** on the concept of human 'culture', the **problem is** that 'culture' is itself shaped by 'nature'. [Two main clauses joined by only a comma]

Correct Even though the concept of 'nature' depends on the concept of human 'culture', 'culture' is itself shaped by 'nature'. [Subordinate clause plus a main clause]

Correct The concept of 'nature' depends on the concept of human 'culture', but 'culture' is itself shaped by 'nature'. [Two main clauses joined by a comma and coordinating conjunction]

The word *however* produces some of the most common comma splice errors. *However* usually functions to begin a main clause, and when it does it should be preceded by a semicolon rather than a comma.

Incorrect The foreign affairs minister repeatedly vowed that the government wasn't choosing a side between the two countries embroiled in conflict, **however** the developing foreign policy suggested otherwise.

Correct The foreign affairs minister repeatedly vowed that the government wasn't choosing a side between the two countries embroiled in conflict**; however,** the developing foreign policy suggested otherwise. [Two main clauses joined by a semicolon]

Remember: Don't use a comma as a full stop.

2. Change the comma to a semicolon.

A semicolon indicates a close connection between two main clauses.

> It didn't matter that I worked in a windowless room for 40 hours a ~~week,~~ *week;* on the Web I was exploring and learning more about distant people and places than I ever had before.

3. Insert a coordinating conjunction.

Other comma splices can be repaired by inserting a coordinating conjunction (*and, but, or, nor, so, yet, for*) to indicate the relationship between the two main clauses. The coordinating conjunction must be preceded by a comma.

> Digital technologies have intensified a global culture that affects us daily in large and small ways, **yet** their impact remains poorly understood.

4. Make one of the main clauses a subordinate clause.

If a comma splice includes one main clause that is subordinate to the other, rewrite the sentence using a subordinating conjunction.

> *Because community*
> ~~Community~~ is the vision of a great society trimmed down to the size of a small town, it is a powerful metaphor for real estate developers who sell a mini-utopia along with a house or an apartment.

5. Make one of the main clauses a phrase.

You can also rewrite one of the main clauses as a phrase.

> Community—**the vision of a great society trimmed down to the size of a small town**—is a powerful metaphor for real estate developers who sell a mini-utopia along with a house or an apartment.

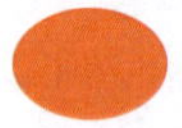

Agreement in the Present Tense

When your verb is in the present tense, agreement in number is straightforward: the subject takes the base form of the verb in all but the third person singular. For example, the verb *walk*, in the present tense, agrees in number with most subjects in its base form.

First person singular	I walk
Second person singular	You walk
First person plural	We walk
Second person plural	You walk
Third person plural	They walk

Third person singular subjects are the exception to this rule. When your subject is in the third person singular (*he*, *it*, *Lucky*, *Lucy*, *Mr Jones*) you need to add *s* or *es* to the base form of the verb.

Third person singular (add *s*)	He walks. It walks. Lucky walks.
Third person singular (add *es*)	Lucy goes. Mr Jones goes.

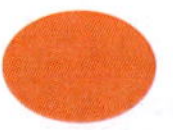

Singular and Plural Subjects

Follow these rules when you have trouble determining whether to use a singular or a plural verb form.

Subjects joined by *and*

When two subjects are joined by *and*, treat them as a compound (plural) subject.

> **The teacher and the solicitor** are headed west to start a commune.

Some compound subjects work together as a single noun and are treated as singular. Although they appear to be compound and therefore plural, these subjects take the singular form of the verb.

Rock and roll remains the devil's music, even in the twenty-first century.

When two nouns linked by *and* are modified by *every* or *each*, these two nouns are likewise treated as one singular subject.

Each night and day brings no new news of you.

An exception to this rule arises when the word *each* follows a compound subject. In these cases, usage varies depending on the number of the direct object.

The army and the navy each have their own planes.

The owl and the pussycat each has a personal claim to fame.

Subjects joined by *or*, *either … or*, or *neither … nor*

When a subject is joined by *or*, *either … or*, or *neither … nor*, make sure the verb agrees with the subject closest to the verb.

SING PLURAL PL
Is it **the sky or the mountains** that are blue?
PLURAL SING SING
Is it **the mountains or the sky** that surrounds us?
PLURAL SING SING
Neither the animals nor the zookeeper knows how to relock the gate.
SING PLURAL PL
Either a dingo or several dogs were howling last night.

Subjects along with another noun

Verbs agree with the subject of a sentence, even when a subject is linked to another noun with a phrase like *as well as*, *along with* or *alongside*. These modifying phrases are usually set off from the main subject with commas.

IGNORE THIS PHRASE
Chicken, alongside various steamed vegetables, is my favourite meal.
IGNORE THIS PHRASE
Besides B.B. King, **John Lee Hooker and Muddy Waters** are my favourite blues artists of all time.

COMMON ERRORS

Subjects separated from verbs

The most common agreement errors occur when words come between the subject and the verb. These intervening words don't affect subject–verb agreement. To ensure that you use the correct verb form, identify the subject and the verb. Ignore any phrases that come between them.

Incorrect **Students** at inner-city Sydney High **reads** more than suburban students.

Correct **Students** at inner-city Sydney High **read** more than suburban students.

Students is plural and *read* is plural; subject and verb agree.

Incorrect **The whale shark**, the largest of all sharks, **feed** on plankton.

Correct **The whale shark**, the largest of all sharks, **feeds** on plankton.

The plural noun *sharks* that appears between the subject *the whale shark* and the verb *feeds* doesn't change the number of the subject. The subject is singular and the verb is singular. Subject and verb agree.

Remember: When you check for subject–verb agreement, identify the subject and the verb. Ignore any words that come between them.

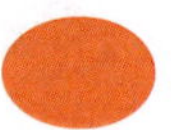

Indefinite Pronouns as Subjects

The choice of a singular or plural pronoun is determined by the **antecedent**—the noun that pronoun refers to. Indefinite pronouns, such as *some, few, all, someone, everyone* and *each,* often don't refer to identifiable subjects; hence they have no antecedents. Most indefinite pronouns are singular and agree with the singular forms of verbs. Some, like *both* and *many,* are always plural and agree with the plural forms of verbs. Other indefinite pronouns are variable and can agree with either singular or plural verb forms, depending on the context of the sentence.

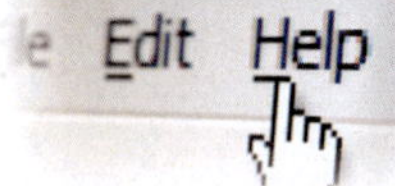

COMMON ERRORS

Agreement errors using *each*

When a pronoun is singular, its verb must be singular. A common stumbling block to this rule is the pronoun *each*. *Each* is always treated as a singular pronoun in academic writing. When *each* stands alone, the choice is easy to make:

Incorrect **Each** **are** an outstanding student.

Correct **Each** **is** an outstanding student.

But when *each* is modified by a phrase that includes a plural noun, the choice of a singular verb form becomes less obvious:

Incorrect **Each** of the girls **are** fit.

Correct **Each** of the girls **is** fit.

Incorrect **Each** of our dogs **get** a present.

Correct **Each** of our dogs **gets** a present.

Remember: *Each* is always singular.

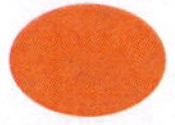

Collective Nouns as Subjects

Collective nouns refer to groups (*audience, class, committee, crowd, family, government, group, jury, public, team*). When members of a group are considered as a unit, use singular verbs and singular pronouns.

> The **crowd** **is** unusually quiet at the moment, but **it** will get noisy soon.

When members of a group are considered as individuals, use plural verbs and plural pronouns.

> The **faculty** **have their** differing opinions on how to address the problems caused by reduced government support.

Sometimes collective nouns can be singular in one context and plural in another. Writers must decide which verb form to use based on sentence context.

The **number** of people who live in the inner city **is** increasing.

A **number** of people **are** moving into the inner city from the suburbs.

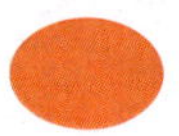

Inverted Word Order

In English a sentence's subject usually comes before the verb: *The nights are tender*. Sometimes, however, you will come across a sentence with inverted word order: *Tender are the nights*. Here the subject of the sentence, *nights*, comes after the verb, *are*. Writers use inverted word order most often in forming questions. The statement *Cats are friendly* becomes a question when you invert the subject and the verb: *Are cats friendly?* Writers also use inverted word order for added emphasis or for style considerations.

Don't be confused by inverted word order. Locate the subject of your sentence, then make sure your verb agrees with that subject.

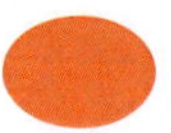

Amounts, Numbers and Pairs

Subjects that describe amounts of money, time, distance or measurement are singular and require singular verbs.

Three days is never long enough to unwind.

Some subjects, such as courses of study, academic specialisations, illnesses and even some nations, are treated as singular subjects even though their names end in *-s* or *-es*. For example, *economics*, *news*, *ethics*, *measles* and *the Philippines* all end in *-s* but are all singular subjects.

Economics is a rich field of study.

Other subjects require a plural verb form even though they refer to single items such as *jeans*, *slacks*, *glasses*, *scissors* and *tweezers*. These items are all pairs.

My **glasses are** scratched.

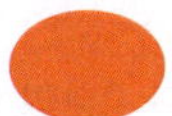

Basic Verb Forms

Almost all verbs in English have five possible forms. The exception is the verb *be*. Regular verbs follow this basic pattern:

Base form	Third person singular	Past tense	Past participle	Present participle
jump	jumps	jumped	jumped	jumping
like	likes	liked	liked	liking
talk	talks	talked	talked	talking
wish	wishes	wished	wished	wishing

Base form

The base form of the verb is the one you find listed in the dictionary. This form indicates an action or condition in the present.

I **like** Darwin in June.

Third person singular

Third person singular subjects include *he*, *she*, *it*, and the nouns they replace, as well as other pronouns, including *someone*, *anybody* and *everything*. Present tense verbs in the third person singular end with *s* or *es*.

Ms Nessan **speaks** in riddles.

Past tense

The past tense describes an action or condition that occurred in the past. For most verbs, the past tense is formed by adding *d* or *ed* to the base form of the verb.

She **inhaled** the night air.

Many verbs, however, have irregular past tense forms. (See Section 24b.)

Past participle

The past participle is used with *have* to form verbs in the perfect tense, with *be* to form verbs in the passive voice (see Section 18a), and to form adjectives derived from verbs.

Past perfect	They **had** **gone** to the supermarket prematurely.
Passive	The book **was** **written** thirty years before it **was** **published**.
Adjective	In the eighties, **teased** hair was all the rage.

COMMON ERRORS

Missing verb endings

Verb endings are not always pronounced in speech, especially in some dialects of English. It is also easy to omit these endings when you are writing quickly. Spelling checkers won't mark these errors, so you have to find them while proofreading.

Incorrect	Jeremy **feel** as if he's catching a cold.
Correct	Jeremy **feels** as if he's catching a cold.
Incorrect	Sarah **hope** she would get the day off.
Correct	Sarah **hoped** she would get the day off.

Remember: Check verbs carefully for missing *s* or *es* endings in the present tense and missing *d* or *ed* endings in the past tense.

Present participle

The present participle functions in one of three ways. Used with an auxiliary verb, it can describe a continuing action. The present participle can also function as a noun, known as a **gerund**, or as an adjective. The present participle is formed by adding *ing* to the base form of a verb.

Present participle	Wild camels **are** **competing** for limited food resources.
Gerund	**Sailing** around the Cape of Good Hope is rumoured to bring good luck.
Adjective	We looked for shells in the **ebbing** tide.

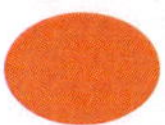

Irregular Verbs

A verb is **regular** when its past and past participle forms are created by adding *ed* or *d* to the base form. If this rule doesn't apply, the verb is considered an **irregular** verb. Here are selected common irregular verbs and their basic conjugations.

Base form	Past tense	Past participle
be (is, am, are)	was, were	been
become	became	become
bring	brought	brought
come	came	come
do	did	done
get	got	got or gotten
have	had	had
go	went	gone
know	knew	known
see	saw	seen

COMMON ERRORS

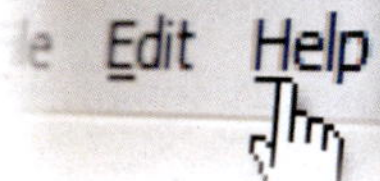

Past tense forms of irregular verbs

The past tense and past participle forms of irregular verbs are often confused. The most frequent error is using a past tense form instead of the past participle with *had*.

Incorrect She had never **rode** a horse before.

Correct She had never **ridden** a horse before.

Incorrect He had **saw** many crocodiles in Kakadu.

Correct He had **seen** many crocodiles in Kakadu.

Remember: Change any past tense verbs preceded by *had* to past participles.

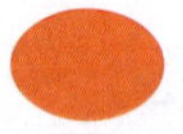

Transitive and Intransitive Verbs

Lay/lie, *set/sit* and *raise/rise*

Do your house keys lay or lie on the kitchen table? Does a book set or sit on the shelf? *Raise/rise*, *lay/lie* and *set/sit* are transitive/intransitive verb pairs that writers frequently confuse. **Transitive verbs** take direct objects—nouns that receive the action of the verb. **Intransitive verbs** act in sentences that lack direct objects.

Transitive Henry **sets** the book [direct object, the book being set] on the shelf.

Intransitive Henry **sits** down to read the book.

The following charts list the trickiest pairs of transitive and intransitive verbs and the correct forms for each verb tense. Pay special attention to *lay* and *lie*, which are irregular.

	lay (put something down)	**lie (recline)**
Present	lay, lays	lie, lies
Present participle	laying	lying
Past	laid	lay
Past participle	laid	lain

Transitive When you complete your test, please **lay** your pencil [direct object, the thing being laid down] on the desk.

Intransitive The *Titanic* **lies** upright in two pieces at a depth of 4000 metres.

	raise (elevate something)	rise (get up)
Present	raise, raises	rise, rises
Present participle	raising	rising
Past	raised	rose
Past participle	raised	risen

Transitive We **raise** our glasses [direct object, the things being raised] to toast Uncle Han.

Intransitive The sun **rises** over the bay.

	set (place something)	sit (take a seat)
Present	set, sets	sit, sits
Present participle	setting	sitting
Past	set	sat
Past participle	set	sat

Transitive Every morning Stanley **sets** two dollars [direct object, the things being set] on the table to tip the waiter.

Intransitive I **sit** in the front seat if it's available.

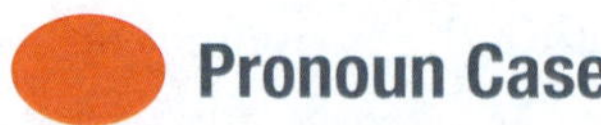

Pronoun Case

Subjective pronouns function as the subjects of sentences. Objective pronouns function as direct or indirect objects. Possessive pronouns indicate ownership.

Subjective pronouns	Objective pronouns	Possessive pronouns
I	me	my, mine
we	us	our, ours
you	you	your, yours
he	him	his
she	her	her, hers
it	it	its
they	them	their, theirs
who	whom	whose

Pronouns in compound phrases

Picking the right pronoun can sometimes be confusing when the pronoun appears in a compound phrase.

> If we work together, you and **me** can get the job done quickly.
>
> If we work together, you and **I** can get the job done quickly.

Which is correct—*me* or *I*? Removing the other pronoun usually makes the choice clear.

Incorrect **Me** can get the job done quickly.

Correct **I** can get the job done quickly.

We and *us* before nouns

Another pair of pronouns that can cause difficulty is *we* and *us* before nouns.

Us friends must stick together.

We friends must stick together.

Which is correct—*us* or *we*? Removing the noun indicates the correct choice.

Incorrect	**Us** must stick together.
Correct	**We** must stick together.

Who versus *whom*

Choosing between *who* and *whom* is often difficult, even for experienced writers. The distinction between *who* and *whom* is disappearing from spoken language. *Who* is more often used in spoken language, even when *whom* is correct.

COMMON ERRORS

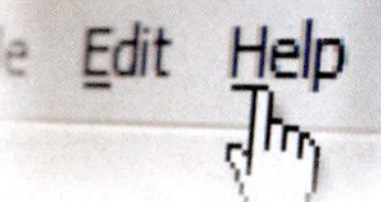

Who or Whom

In writing, the distinction between *who* and *whom* is still often observed. *Who* and *whom* follow the same rules as other pronouns: *Who* is the subject pronoun; *whom* is the object pronoun. If you are dealing with an object, *whom* is the correct choice.

Incorrect	**Who** did you send the letter to?
	Who did you give the present to?
Correct	To **whom** did you send the letter?
	Whom did you give the present to?

Who is always the right choice for the subject pronoun.

Correct	**Who** gave you the present?
	Who brought the beers?

COMMON ERRORS

If you are uncertain of which one to use, try substituting *she* and *her* or *he* and *him*.

Incorrect You sent the letter to **she [who]**?

Correct You sent the letter to **her [whom]**?

Incorrect **Him [Whom]** gave you the present?

Correct **He [Who]** gave you the present?

Remember: *Who* = subject; *whom* = object.

Whoever versus *whomever*

With the rule regarding *who* and *whom* in mind, you can distinguish between *whoever* and *whomever*. Which is correct?

Her warmth touched **whoever** she met.

Her warmth touched **whomever** she met.

In this sentence the pronoun functions as the direct object in its own clause: she met whomever. Thus *whomever* is the correct choice.

Pronouns in comparisons

When you write a sentence using a comparison that includes *than* or *as* followed by a pronoun, usually you will have to think about which pronoun is correct. Which of the following is correct?

Vimala is a faster swimmer than **him.**

Vimala is a faster swimmer than **he.**

The test that will give you the correct answer is to add the verb that finishes the sentence—in this case, *is*.

Incorrect Vimala is a faster swimmer than **him is.**

Correct Vimala is a faster swimmer than **he is.**

Adding the verb makes the correct choice evident.

Possessive pronouns

Possessive pronouns are confusing at times because possessive nouns are formed with apostrophes, but possessive pronouns don't require apostrophes. Pronouns that use apostrophes are always **contractions**.

It's = It is

Who's = Who is

They're = They are

The test for whether to use an apostrophe is to determine whether the pronoun is possessive or a contraction. The most confusing pair is *its* and *it's*.

Incorrect	**Its** a sure thing she will be elected. [Contraction needed]
Correct	**It's** a sure thing she will be elected. [It is a sure thing.]
Incorrect	The dog lost **it's** collar. [Possessive needed]
Correct	The dog lost **its** collar.

Possessive pronouns before *-ing* verbs

Pronouns that modify an *-ing* verb (called a *gerund*) or an *-ing* verb phrase (*gerund phrase*) should appear in the possessive.

Incorrect	The odds of **you** making the team are excellent.
Correct	The odds of **your** making the team are excellent.

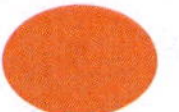

Pronoun Agreement

Because pronouns usually replace or refer to other nouns, they must match those nouns in number and gender. The noun that the pronoun replaces is called its **antecedent**. If pronoun and antecedent match, they are in **agreement**. When a pronoun is close to the antecedent, usually there is no problem.

Maria forgot **her** coat.

The band **members** collected **their** uniforms.

Pronoun agreement errors often happen when pronouns and the nouns they replace are separated by several words.

Incorrect

The **players**, exhausted from the double-overtime game, picked up **his** tracksuit and walked towards the club rooms.

Correct

The **players**, exhausted from the double-overtime game, picked up **their** tracksuits and walked towards the club rooms.

Careful writers make sure that pronouns match their antecedents.

COMMON ERRORS

Indefinite pronouns

Indefinite pronouns (such as *anybody*, *anything*, *each*, *either*, *everybody*, *everything*, *neither*, *none*, *somebody*, *something*) refer to unspecified people or things. Most take singular pronouns.

Incorrect Everybody can choose **their** flatmates.

Correct Everybody can choose **his or her** flatmate.

Correct alternative All students can choose **their** flatmates.

A few indefinite pronouns (*all*, *any*, *either*, *more*, *most*, *neither*, *none*, *some*) can take either singular or plural pronouns.

Correct **Some** of the shipment was damaged when **it** became overheated.

Correct **All** thought **they** should have a good seat at the concert.

A few pronouns are always plural (*few*, *many*, *several*).

Correct **Several** want refunds.

Remember: Words that begin with *any*, *some* and *every* are usually singular.

Collective nouns

Collective nouns (such as *audience, class, committee, crowd, family, herd, jury, team*) can be singular or plural depending on whether the emphasis is on the group or on its individual members.

Correct The **committee** was unanimous in **its** decision.

Correct The **committee** put **their** opinions ahead of the goals of the unit.

COMMON ERRORS

Pronoun agreement with compound antecedents

Antecedents joined by *and* take plural pronouns.

Correct *Moncef and Driss* practised **their** music.

Exception: When compound antecedents are preceded by *each* or *every*, use a singular pronoun.

Correct **Every male cardinal and warbler** arrives before the female to define **its** territory.

When compound antecedents are connected by *or* or *nor*, the pronoun agrees with the antecedent closer to it.

Incorrect **Either the Ross twins or Angela** should bring **their** CDs.

Correct **Either the Ross twins or Angela** should bring **her** CDs.

Better **Either Angela or the Ross twins** should bring **their** CDs.

When you put the plural *twins* last, the correct choice becomes the plural pronoun *their*.

Remember:

1. **Use plural pronouns for antecedents joined by *and*.**
2. **Use singular pronouns for antecedents preceded by *each* or *every*.**
3. **Use a pronoun that agrees with the nearest antecedent when compound antecedents are joined by *or* or *nor*.**

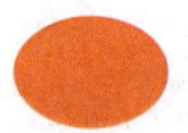

Avoid Sexist Pronouns

English doesn't have a neutral singular pronoun for a group of mixed genders or a person of unknown gender. Referring to a group of mixed genders using male pronouns is unacceptable to many people. Unless the school in the following example is all male, many readers would object to the use of *his*.

Sexist **Each student** must select **his** courses using the online registration system.

One strategy is to use *her or his* or *his or her* instead of *his*.

Correct **Each student** must select **his or her** courses using the online registration system.

Often you can avoid using *his or her* by changing the noun to the plural form.

Better **All students** must select **their** courses using the online registration system.

In some cases, however, using *his or her* is necessary.

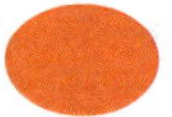

Vague Reference

Pronouns can sometimes refer to more than one noun, thus confusing readers.

> The **coach** rushed past the injured **player** to yell at the **referee**. **She** was hit in the face by a stray elbow.

You have to guess which person *she* refers to—the coach, the player or the referee. Sometimes you cannot even guess the antecedent of a pronoun.

> The new subdivision destroyed the last remaining habitat for wildlife within the city limits. **They** have ruined our city with their unchecked greed.

To whom does *they* refer? the mayor and city council? the developers? the people who live in the subdivision? or all of the above?

Pronouns should never leave the reader guessing about antecedents. If different nouns can be confused as the antecedent, then the ambiguity should be clarified.

Vague Siham's pet python crawled across Tonya's foot. **She** was mortified.

Better When Siham's pet python crawled across Tonya's foot, **Siham** was mortified.

COMMON ERRORS

Vague use of this

Always use a noun immediately after *this*, *that*, *these*, *those* and *some*.

Vague Enrique asked Meg to remove the viruses on his computer. **This** was a bad idea.

Was it a bad idea for Enrique to ask Meg because she was insulted? Because she didn't know how? Because removing viruses would destroy some of Enrique's files?

Better Enrique asked Meg to remove the viruses on his computer. **This imposition** on Meg's time was a bad idea.

Remember: Ask yourself 'this *what*?' and add the noun that *this* refers to.

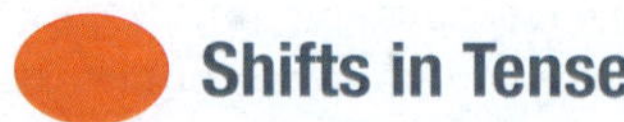

Shifts in Tense

Appropriate shifts in verb tense

Changes in verb tense are sometimes necessary to indicate a shift in time.

Past to future

PAST TENSE / FUTURE TENSE / PRESENT TENSE

Because Oda **won** the lottery, she **will quit** her job at the hospital as soon as her supervisor **finds** **a** qualified replacement.

Inappropriate shifts in verb tense

Be careful to avoid confusing your reader with shifts in verb tense.

Incorrect

PRESENT TENSE / PAST TENSE

While Brazil **looks** to ecotourism to fund rainforest preservation, other South American nations **relied** on foreign aid and conservation efforts.

The shift from present tense (*looks*) to past tense (*relied*) is confusing. Correct the mistake by putting both verbs in the present tense.

Correct

PRESENT TENSE / PRESENT TENSE

While Brazil **looks** to ecotourism to fund rainforest preservation, other South American nations **rely** on foreign aid and conservation efforts.

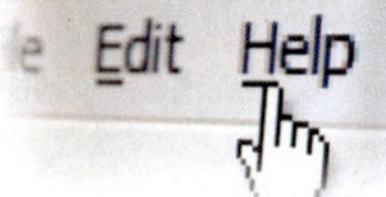

COMMON ERRORS

Unnecessary tense shift

Notice the tense shift in the following example.

Incorrect In May 2000 the 'I Love You' virus **crippled** the computer systems of many major companies and **irritated** millions of private computer users. As the virus **generates** millions of emails and **erases** millions of computer files, many companies **are** forced to shut down their clogged email systems.

The second sentence shifts unnecessarily to the present tense, confusing the reader. Did the 'I Love You' virus have its heyday a decade ago, or is it still wreaking havoc now? Changing the verbs in the second sentence to the past tense eliminates the confusion.

Correct In May 2000 the 'I Love You' virus **crippled** the computer systems of many major companies and **irritated** millions of private computer users. As the virus **generated** millions of emails and **erased** millions of computer files, many companies **were** forced to shut down their clogged email systems.

Remember: Shift verb tense only when you are referring to different time periods.

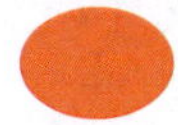

Shifts in Mood

Verbs can be categorised into three moods—indicative, imperative and subjunctive—defined by the functions they serve.

Indicative verbs state facts, opinions and questions.

Fact Qantas **plans** to boost its domestic seat capacity to make up for losses incurred during the global financial crisis.

Imperative verbs make commands, give advice and make requests.

Command **Make up** for losses incurred during the global financial crisis by boosting domestic seat capacity.

Subjunctive verbs express wishes, unlikely or untrue situations, hypothetical situations, requests with *that* clauses, and suggestions.

Unlikely or untrue situation If improving profitability **were** as simple as merely increasing seat capacity, Qantas would be assured of making up for losses incurred during the global financial crisis.

Be careful not to shift from one mood to another in mid-sentence.

Incorrect If Qantas **were** to boost its domestic seat capacity, it **is** difficult for other airlines to maintain market share.

The sudden shift from subjunctive to indicative mood in this sentence is confusing. Is it difficult for the other airlines to maintain market share now, or is difficulty in maintaining market share a likely result of Qantas boosting its seat capacity? Revise the sentence to keep both verbs in the subjunctive.

Correct If Qantas **were** to boost its domestic seat capacity, it **would be** difficult for other airlines to maintain market share.

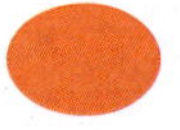

Shifts in Voice

Watch for unintended shifts from active voice (*I ate the biscuits*) to passive voice (*the biscuits were eaten*).

Incorrect The sudden storm **toppled** several trees and numerous windows **were shattered.**

The unexpected shift from active voice (*toppled*) to passive voice (*were shattered*) forces readers to wonder whether it was the sudden storm, or something else, that broke the windows.

Correct The sudden storm **toppled** several trees and **shattered** numerous windows.

Revising the sentence to eliminate the shift to passive voice (see Section 18a) also improves its parallel structure (see 20c).

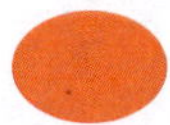

Shifts in Person and Number

Sudden shifts from third person (*he*, *she*, *it*, *one*) to first (*I*, *we*) or second (*you*) are confusing to readers and often indicate a writer's uncertainty about how to address a reader. We often make such shifts in spoken English, but in formal writing shifts in person need to be recognised and corrected.

Incorrect When **one** is reading a magazine, **you** often see several different type fonts used on a single page.

The shift from third person to second person in this sentence is confusing.

Correct When reading a magazine **you** often see several different type fonts used on a single page.

Shifts from singular to plural subjects (see Section 23b) within a single sentence also confuse readers.

Incorrect Administrators often make more money than **lecturers**, but only **a lecturer** has frequent contact with students.

Correct Administrators often make more money than **lecturers**, but only **lecturers** have frequent contact with students.

The revised sentence eliminates a distracting and unnecessary shift from plural to singular.

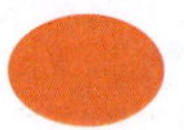

Choose the Correct Modifier

Modifiers come in two varieties: adjectives and adverbs. The same words can function as adjectives or adverbs, depending on what they modify.

Adjectives modify

nouns—*iced* tea, *fast* runner
pronouns—He is *brash*.

Adverbs modify

verbs—*barely* reach, drive *carefully*
adjectives—*truly* brave activist, *shockingly* red lipstick
other adverbs—*not* soon forget, *very* well
clauses—*Honestly*, I find ballet boring.

Adjectives answer the questions *Which one? How many?* and *What kind?* Adverbs answer the questions *How often? To what extent? When? Where? How?* and *Why?*

Use the correct forms of comparatives and superlatives

Comparative modifiers weigh one thing against another. They either end in *er* or are preceded by *more.*

Road bikes are **faster** on bitumen than mountain bikes.

The **more courageous** juggler tossed flaming torches.

Superlative modifiers compare three or more items. They either end in *est* or are preceded by *most.*

May and June are the **hottest** months in New Delhi.

Wounded animals are the **most ferocious**.

Some frequently used comparatives and superlatives are irregular. The following list can help you become familiar with them.

Adjective	Comparative	Superlative
good	better	best
bad	worse	worst
little (amount)	less	least
many, much	more	most

Adverb	Comparative	Superlative
well	better	best
badly	worse	worst

Don't use both a suffix (*er* or *est*) and *more* or *most.*

Incorrect The service at Jane's Restaurant is **more slower** than the service at Alphonso's.

Correct The service at Jane's Restaurant is **slower** than the service at Alphonso's.

Absolute modifiers are words that represent an unvarying condition and thus aren't subject to the degrees that comparative and superlative constructions convey. Common absolute modifiers include *complete*, *ultimate* and *unique. Unique*, for example, means 'one of a kind'. There is nothing else like it. Thus something cannot be *very unique* or *totally unique*. It is either unique or it isn't. Absolute modifiers shouldn't be modified by comparatives (*more* + modifier or modifier + *er*) or superlatives (*most* + modifier or modifier + *est*).

Double negatives

In English, as in mathematics, two negatives equal a positive. Avoid using two negative words in one sentence, or you will end up saying the opposite of what you mean. The following are negative words that you should avoid doubling up:

barely	nobody	nothing
hardly	none	scarcely
neither	no one	

Incorrect, double negative	**Barely no one** noticed that the pop star lip-synched during the whole performance.
Correct, single negative	**Barely anyone** noticed that the pop star lip-synched during the whole performance.
Incorrect, double negative	When the minister asked if anyone had objections to the marriage, **nobody** said **nothing**.
Correct, single negative	When the minister asked if anyone had objections to the marriage, **nobody** said **anything**.

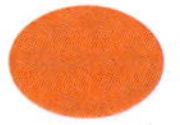

Place Adjectives Carefully

As a general rule, the closer you place a modifier to the word it modifies, the less it is likely that you will confuse your reader.

Confusing	**Watching from the ground below**, the eagles circled high above the observers.

Are the eagles watching from the ground below? You can fix the problem by putting the modified subject immediately after the modifier or placing the modifier next to the modified subject.

Better	The eagles circled high above the **observers** **who were watching from the ground below**.
Better	**Watching from the ground below**, the **observers** saw eagles circling high above them.

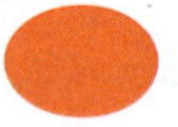

Place Adverbs Carefully

Single-word adverbs and adverbial clauses and phrases can usually sit comfortably either before or after the words they modify.

Dimitri **quietly** **walked** down the hall.

Dimitri **walked** **quietly** down the hall.

Conjunctive adverbs—*also, however, instead, likewise, then, therefore, thus* and others—are adverbs that show how ideas relate to one another. They prepare a reader for contrasts, exceptions, additions, conclusions and other shifts in an argument. Conjunctive adverbs can usually fit well into more than one place in the sentence. In the following example, *however* could fit in three different places.

Between two main clauses

Professional football players earn very high salaries; **however,** they pay for their wealth with lifetimes of chronic pain and debilitating injuries.

Within second main clause

Professional football players earn very high salaries; they pay for their wealth, **however,** with lifetimes of chronic pain and debilitating injuries.

At end of second main clause

Professional football players earn very high salaries; they pay for their wealth with lifetimes of chronic pain and debilitating injuries **however**.

Subordinating conjunctions—words such as *after*, *although*, *because*, *if*, *since*, *than*, *that*, *though*, *when* and *where*—often begin **adverb clauses**. Notice that we can place adverb clauses with subordinating conjunctions either before or after the word(s) being modified:

After someone in the audience yelled, he **forgot** the lyrics.

He **forgot** the lyrics **after someone in the audience yelled**.

COMMON ERRORS

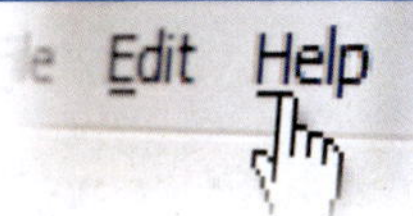

Placement of limiting modifiers

Words such as *almost*, *even*, *hardly*, *just*, *merely*, *nearly*, *not*, *only* and *simply* are called limiting modifiers. Although people often play fast and loose with their placement in everyday speech, limiting modifiers should always go immediately before the word or words they modify in your writing. Like other limiting modifiers, *only* should be placed immediately before the word it modifies.

COMMON ERRORS

Incorrect The Gross Domestic Product **only** gives one indicator of economic growth.

Correct The Gross Domestic Product gives **only** one indicator of economic growth.

The word *only* modifies *one* in this sentence, not *Gross Domestic Product.*

Remember: Place limiting modifiers immediately before the word(s) they modify.

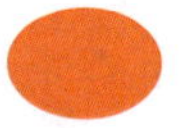

Hyphens with Compound Modifiers

When to hyphenate

Hyphenate a compound modifier that precedes a noun.

When a compound modifier precedes a noun, you should usually hyphenate the modifier. A **compound modifier** consists of words that join together as a unit to modify a noun.

middle-class values   self-fulfilling prophecy

Hyphenate a phrase when it is used as a modifier that precedes a noun.

all-you-can-eat buffet   step-by-step instructions

Hyphenate the prefixes *pro-*, *anti-*, *post-*, *pre-*, *neo-* and *mid-* before proper nouns and some common nouns.

neo-Nazi racism   mid-Pacific storms

Hyphenate a compound modifier with a number when it precedes a noun.

eighteenth-century drama   one-way street

When not to hyphenate

Don't hyphenate a compound modifier that follows a noun.

The tutor's approach is student centred.

Don't hyphenate compound modifiers when the first word is *very* or ends in *ly*.

newly recorded data very cold day

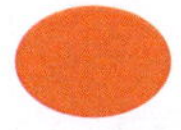

Revise Dangling Modifiers

Some modifiers are ambiguous because they could apply to more than one word or clause. Dangling modifiers are ambiguous for the opposite reason; they don't have a word to modify. In such cases the modifier is usually an introductory clause or phrase. What is being modified should immediately follow the phrase, but in the following sentence it is absent.

After bowling a perfect game, Surfside Bowling Alley hung Marco's photo on the wall.

You can eliminate a dangling modifier in two ways:

1. Insert the noun or pronoun being modified immediately after the introductory modifying phrase.

   After bowling a perfect game, **Marco** was honoured by having his photo hung on the wall at Surfside Bowling Alley.

2. Rewrite the introductory phrase as an introductory clause to include the noun or pronoun.

   After **Marco** bowled a perfect game, Surfside Bowling Alley hung his photo on the wall.

COMMON ERRORS

Dangling modifiers

A dangling modifier doesn't seem to modify anything in a sentence; it dangles, unconnected to the word or words it presumably is intended to modify. Frequently, it produces funny results:

When still a girl, my father took up parachuting.

It sounds like *father* was once a girl. The problem is that the subject, *I*, is missing:

When I was still a girl, my father took up parachuting.

Remember: Modifiers should be clearly connected to the words they modify, especially at the beginning of sentences.

Nouns

Perhaps the most troublesome conventions for non-native speakers are those that guide usage of the common articles *the*, *a* and *an*. To understand how articles work in English, you must first understand how the language uses nouns.

Kinds of nouns

There are two basic kinds of nouns. A **proper noun** begins with a capital letter and names a unique person, place or thing: *Ian Thorpe*, *Indonesia*, *Melbourne Cricket Ground*.

The other basic kind of noun is called a **common noun**. Common nouns don't name a unique person, place or thing: *man*, *country*, *sportsground*.

Countable and uncountable nouns

Common nouns can be classified as either *countable* or *uncountable*. **Countable nouns** can be made plural, usually by adding *-s* (*finger*, *fingers*) or by using their plural forms (*person*, *people*; *datum*, *data*). **Uncountable nouns** cannot be counted directly and cannot take the plural form (*information*, but not *informations*; *garbage*, but not *garbages*). Some nouns can be either countable or uncountable, depending on how they are used. *Hair* can refer to either a strand of hair, where it serves as a countable noun, or a mass of hair, where it becomes an uncountable noun.

COMMON ERRORS

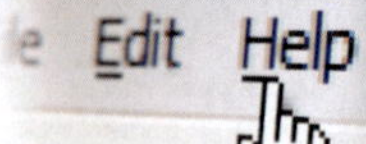

Singular and plural forms of countable nouns

Countable nouns are simpler to quantify than uncountable nouns. But remember that English requires you to state both singular and plural forms of nouns explicitly. Look at the following sentences.

Incorrect The three **cyclist** shaved their **leg** before the big race.

Correct The three **cyclists** shaved their **legs** before the big race.

Remember: English requires you to use plural forms of countable nouns even if a plural number is otherwise indicated.

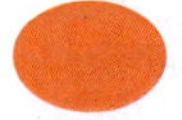

Articles

Articles indicate that a noun is about to appear, and they clarify what the noun refers to. There are only two kinds of articles in English, definite and indefinite:

1. **the:** *The* is a **definite article**, meaning that it refers to (1) a specific object already known to the reader, (2) one about to be made known to the reader, or (3) a unique object.
2. **a, an:** The **indefinite articles** *a* and *an* refer to an object whose specific identity isn't known to the reader. The only difference between *a* and *an* is that *a* is used before a consonant sound (*man, friend, yellow*), while *an* is used before a vowel sound (*animal, enemy, orange*).

COMMON ERRORS

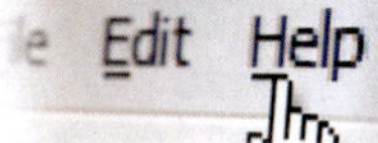

Articles with countable and uncountable nouns

Knowing how to distinguish between countable and uncountable nouns can help you decide which article to use. Uncountable nouns are never used with the indefinite articles *a* or *an*.

Incorrect Maria jumped into **a** water.

Correct Maria jumped into **the** water.

No articles are used with uncountable and plural countable nouns when you wish to state something that has a general application.

Incorrect **The** water is a precious natural resource.

Correct Water is a precious natural resource.

Remember:

1. **Uncountable nouns are never used with *a* and *an*.**
2. **Uncountable and plural nouns used to make general statements don't take articles.**

12 The purpose of assessment

The purpose of assessment is to determine student understanding of specific topics within a course and to enhance student learning. There are different methods of assessment: formative and summative.

Formative assessments are designed primarily to improve learning while summative assessments are designed to judge learning (Crisp, 2012, p. 33). All courses will have a mix of formative and summative assessment

All assessments should align to the program, course objectives and topic objectives and the University Graduate Qualities. This is made explicit in the course outline for each topic and is pointed out to students and explained at the commencement of each course.

Assessments within courses can take many forms:

- Written assessment on a topic- the traditional essay
- Physical assessment of competencies, skills
- Online quizzes- multiple choice questions for example
- Case study analysis
- Online interactive assessments
- Oral vivas
- Examinations

It is important to note that all assessments are designed as vehicles for knowledge transfer: theoretical knowledge to practice.

13 How to read and understand the assessment task

It is important for students to know how to read and understand the assessment task. See the strategies for effective reading above. The URL below will take you to the Learning & Teaching Unit's information about assessments.

http://resource.unisa.edu.au/course/view.php?id=3633&topic=4

Key points to note with assessment tasks:

- Subject, topic, due date.
- Read the instructions carefully
- If you have any questions about the assessment always ask your lecturer and NOT ANOTHER STUDENT.

14 Writing for assessment

Before submitting your written assessment you should review what you have written. Check for spelling errors, grammar and finally sense making. Does what you have written make sense. (Word has a Spell & Grammar check function that should be used). Faigley (2013 p.17) provides the following review questions:

- Does your assignment meet the assignment requirements?
- Does your writing have a clear focus?
- Have you addressed the main points coherently?
- Do you need to rearrange sections of the paper?
- Have you considered your reader's perspectives on the topic?
- Does your conclusion summarise the main points

For all students writing for academic assessment can be quite daunting. Being able to write for academic assessment is an essential skill/competency all students need to develop. An important part of writing for academic success is reading and understanding the marking criteria developed for a particular assignment. It is also an opportunity for you to practice your critical thinking skills interpreting the marking criteria. The next page shows a table of marking criteria taken from Ragusa (2012, p. 148)

Assessment marking criteria exemplar

Marking criteria
Essays will be assessed on the following points:

1. Knowledge of topic. Have the main issues relating to the topic been understood and covered?
2. Application of sociological theory. Have the theories, concepts and subject material been applied to the issue or has a descriptive/ narrative account only been written?
3. Use of pertinent examples and relevant evidence. Have the assertions made and conclusions drawn been adequately supported by reliable and valid evidence?
4. Critical analysis. Have the ideas and data been synthesised and analysed instead of merely collated and rewritten?
5. Quality and range of references. Have all the required readings been read and included and are the independently obtained resources of good quality, appropriately used and cited?
6. Clarity, structure and presentation. Is the essay clear, concise, well organised, unified and coherent? Is there an introduction, body and conclusion?
7. Creativity, originality and required parts. Is the essay a unique expression of thought? Has the author made a novel insight into the issues or regurgitated already published ideas? Have the instructions been followed and all required parts included?

Marks will be lost for:

- inadequate preparation
- not following instructions
- lack of evidence and examples to support arguments
- uncritical summarisation of readings
- inferior references

Source: Charles Sturt University, Subject Outline Introductory Sociology SOC101, Session 2, 2010. Permission to reproduce by Carmen Moran, Charles Sturt University.

15 Marking rubrics

All assessment pieces will be accompanied by a marking rubric and these are available to students. The rubric contains the marking criteria which lecturers use to assess your work. The criteria are listed against the grades for the assessment piece. It is therefore in your best interests to know and understand the criteria underpinning the different grade levels. The rubric is completed by the lecturer and is an element of feedback for a particular assignment. At the back of the book is an example of a marking rubric.

16 E-assessment

Online assessments are an important part of student learning and increasingly used. Online assessments can be quizzes, multiple choice questions; case study analysis. Just as with written assignments it is important to read the instructions provided by teaching staff to successfully complete these assessments. What is important to note about online assessments is that they are timed- that is, they open at a scheduled time on a specified date and close at a scheduled time on a specified date. Students usually only have one opportunity to access the online assessment. That is why it is so important to read the instructions. Failure to follow instructions will result in:

- Lock out from the quiz
- A fail grade for the assessment piece.

Multiple attempts to access the one online assessment is academic misconduct and will be managed as such.

It is timely to remind students that the online environment used by the university has features enabling teaching staff to monitor individual student activity in individual courses.

17 Assessment feedback

Assessment feedback is an important component of teaching and learning. The intent of constructive assessment feedback is to provide students with objective information directly related to their achievements in a particular assessment piece. Areas that could be improved for example writing clearly and for purpose or referencing as well as noting areas that are done well. The assessment feedback should be used as an opportunity for learning improvement by students.

Assessment feedback can be provided through rubrics (a standardised format) or as individual comments on papers (see marking rubric at the back of this book).

18 Time management

Time management is an important consideration when writing assignments simply because assignments have a due date and if you are studying in more than one course/subject you will have many due dates. Good time management enables you to submit your assignments on time and this is appreciated by lecturers who may have a number of papers to mark. It also ensures that your grades are entered in a timely manner especially if you are in your final year and hoping to graduate with your colleagues.

One of the main obstacles to effective time management in this context is procrastination. Procrastination is supported by many excuses such as: 'I do not have time'; or 'I'm too busy, tired'. Students who continually procrastinate often find themselves falling behind in their studies and extending their completion dates which can have economic and social consequences.

All courses have a course calendar with key dates. You should make yourself aware of these dates, especially the assignment due dates and plan your studies around this. The LTU can help students with study time management. The LTU provides students with study planners which may be accessed at: http://w3.unisa.edu.au/languageandlearning/resources/planners.asp

19 Referencing

Referencing is an important part of academic writing. By referencing your work you are demonstrating your ability to source supporting information/evidence for the key issues identified in your paper.

It is important to know what to reference as well as what not to reference.

What not to reference:

- Personal experience information
- Observational informational – observing people in supermarkets
- Historical information- that may be found in multiple reference sources
- Discipline specific information and concepts that exist in multiple reference sources: such as accepted facts Florence Nightingale is regarded as the founder of modern secular nursing
- Common sayings and widespread beliefs: 'saving for rainy day'

(Adapted from Ragusa 2012).

You can access the new Harvard referencing guide here:
http://resource.unisa.edu.au/course/view.php?id=3633&topic=8
and the Learning & Teaching Unit's (LTU) road map to referencing here:
http://roadmap.unisa.edu.au/

20 Academic honesty

Academic honesty means behaving with integrity and within the university's Code of Conduct for students available at http://w3.unisa.edu.au/policies/codes/students/code-of-conduct-for-students.pdf

Academic integrity is an element of academic honesty means presenting all academic (written assessments, exams, online quizzes etc.) work WITHOUT engaging in plagiarism; any form of cheating including emailing to other students/persons screen grabs of university materials (course content; course assessments); lying, tampering, stealing, receiving assistance from any other person/student or using any source of information that is not common knowledge without proper attribution of the source.

Having other people write your assignments or purchasing assignments from online providers is also breaching the Academic Integrity policy and the student code of conduct. Using social media and web based technologies to send university information to other students/persons is also a form of academic dishonesty.

For further information relating to academic integrity go to the University of South Australia's Assessment Policies and Procedures Manual 2013. This manual is reviewed and published annually. It may be accessed at http://w3.unisa.edu.au/policies/manual/2013/APPM_2013-Full_version.pdf

The university uses plagiarism detecting software (TURNITIN) for all written work submitted electronically. Students should be aware of the university's policies relating to academic honesty and these may be found in the university's Assessment Policies & Procedures Manual. This is available electronically in each course.

21 Clinical placements

As a part of your studies you will go out on clinical placements to a number of different health care facilities. A formative assessment of your ability to demonstrate the capacity to translate theoretical knowledge learned at university to the practice setting will be done. This assessment is an important part of your learning experience and uses negotiated learning objectives to measure your performance. Poor behaviour including non-compliance with academic requirements while on clinical placement forms a part of your assessments during this period of your study. These assessments are important because they form a part of the selection process for acceptance into the Transition to Professional Practice Program (TPPP) offered to first year graduate nurses.

Clinical placements commence in first year but it is in the second year of your program that you will be expected to engage with direct patient care activities. In this stage you will be introduced to the clinical practice dimensions of nursing. As a second year student you will be expected to engage in critical thinking and decision making; be able to start making connections between the theoretical components of your course with the practical aspects of your course. For example, you will have to be able to complete head to toe assessments of individual patients and document these. You will be spending more time in the Practice Based Laboratories (PBLs); engage in simulated learning experiences that mimic real life experiences; engage in many more online activities including virtual classrooms. You will also be expected to engage in clinical practice activities that are expected of registered nurses and document this in the format required. You will be expected to describe, analyse and provide justification for your decisions from these activities in writing. Despite the high technological environments you find yourself in - you will be expected to write well without the use of text language.

Other health care disciplines will have their own clinical placement programs and students need to know what their particular program requirements for clinical placement are.

22 Analysing a case study

 Write a Case Study

Case studies are used in a wide range of fields, such as nursing, psychology, business and anthropology. Case studies are narrow in focus, providing a rich, detailed portrait of a specific event or subject.

Elements of a case study

Introduction	Explain the purpose of your study and how or why you selected your subject. Use language appropriate to your discipline, and specify the boundaries of your study.
Methodology	Explain the theories or formal process that guided your observations and analysis during the study.
Observations	Describe the 'case' of the subject under study by writing a narrative, utilising interviews, research and other data to provide as much detail and specificity as possible.
Discussion	Explain how the variables in your case might interact. Don't generalise from your case to a larger context; stay within the limits of what you have observed.
Conclusion	What does all this information add up to? What is implied, suggested or proven by your observations? Situate your analysis in the literature of the discipline. What new questions arise?
References	Using the appropriate format, cite all the outside sources you have used.

What you need to do

- Understand the specific elements of your assignment. Ask your lecturer about what your case study should include.
- Use careful observation and precise, detailed description to provide a complex picture with a narrow focus.
- Write your observations in the form of a narrative, placing yourself in the background (avoid using *I* or *me*).
- Analyse your findings and interpret their possible meanings, but draw your conclusions from the observed facts.

23 Write with power and emphasis

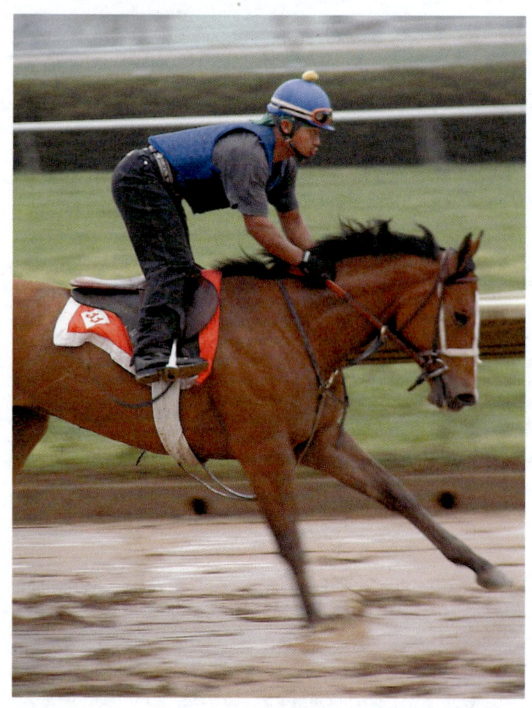

In photographs

You imagine actions when subjects are captured in motion.

In writing

Your readers expect actions to be expressed in verbs:
gallop, canter, trot, run, sprint, dash, bound, thunder, tear away.

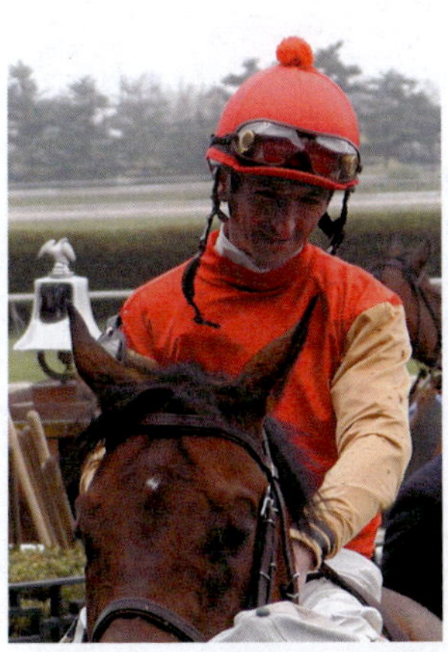

In photographs

Viewers interpret the most prominent person or thing as the subject—what the photograph is about.

In writing

Readers interpret the first person or thing they meet in a sentence as what the sentence is about (the jockey, the horse). They expect that person or thing to perform the action expressed in the verb.

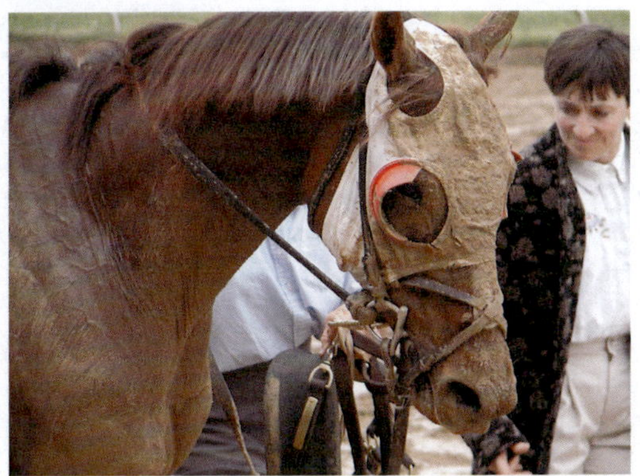

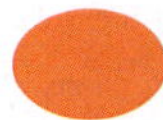

Recognise Active and Passive Voice

In the **active voice** the subject of the sentence is the actor. In the **passive voice** the subject is being acted upon.

Active ***Leonardo da Vinci*** **painted** *Mona Lisa* between 1503 and 1506.

Passive ***Mona Lisa*** **was painted** by Leonardo da Vinci between 1503 and 1506.

To write with power, use the active voice. Observe the difference:

Passive The pear tree in the front yard **was demolished** by the unexpected storm.

Active The unexpected storm **demolished** the pear tree in the front yard.

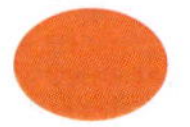

Use Action Verbs

Where are the action words in the following sentences?

> Red hair flying, professional snowboarder and skateboarder Shaun White became a two-time Olympic gold medallist with a record score of 48.4 at the 2010 Winter Olympics. White was a skier before he was five, but became a snowboarder at age six, and by age seven he had become a professional, receiving corporate sponsorships. At age nine, White became friends with professional skateboarder Tony Hawk, who became White's mentor in becoming a professional skateboarder. White is known for accomplishing several 'firsts' in snowboarding, including being the first to land back-to-back double corks and to master a trick called a Cab 7 Melon Grab. He is also the holder of the record for the highest score in the men's halfpipe at the Winter Olympics.

No action words here! The passage describes a series of actions, yet most of the verbs are *is*, *was* and *became*. Think about what the actions are and choose powerful verbs that express those actions.

> Red hair flying, professional snowboarder and skateboarder Shaun White **scored** a 48.4 during the 2010 Winter Olympics and **won** his second gold medal. White **skied** before he was five, but **switched** to snowboarding at age six, and by age seven **received** corporate sponsorships. At age nine, White **befriended** professional skateboarder Tony Hawk, who **mentored** White and **helped** him become a professional skateboarder. White **has accomplished** several 'firsts' in snowboarding, including landing back-to-back double corks and mastering a trick called a Cab 7 Melon Grab. He also **holds** the record for the highest score in the men's halfpipe at the Winter Olympics.

Many sentences contain words that express action, but those words are nouns rather than verbs. Often the nouns can be changed into verbs. For example:

> The arson unit ~~conducted an investigation of~~ **investigated** the mysterious fire.
>
> The committee ~~had a debate over~~ **debated** how best to spend the surplus funds.

Notice that changing nouns into verbs also eliminates unnecessary words.

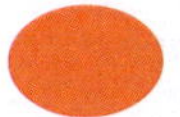

Find Agents

The **agent** is the person or thing that does the action. Powerful writing puts the agents in sentences.

Focus on people

Read the following sentence aloud:

> The use of a MIDI keyboard for playing the song will facilitate capturing it in digital form on a laptop for the subsequent purpose of uploading it to a website.

It sounds dead, doesn't it? Putting people into the sentence makes it come alive:

> By playing the song on a MIDI keyboard, **we** can record the digitised sound on **our** laptop and then upload it to **our** website.

Including people makes your writing more emphatic. Most readers relate better to people than to abstractions. Putting people in your sentences also introduces active verbs because people do things.

Identify characters

If people are not your subject, then keep the focus on other types of characters.

Without characters	The celebration of Australia Day had to be cancelled because of inclement weather.
With characters	A severe **cyclone** forced the **city** to cancel the Australia Day celebration.

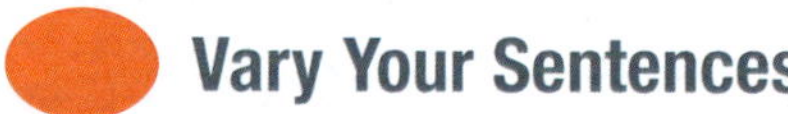

Vary Your Sentences

Read the following passage.

> On the first day Garth, Jim and I paddled fourteen kilometres down Johnstone Strait. We headed down the strait about five more kilometres to Robson Bight. It is a well-known place for seeing dolphins. The Bight is a small bay. We paddled out into the strait so we could see the entire Bight. There were no dolphins to be seen. By this time we were getting tired. We were hungry. The clouds assumed a wintry dark thickness. The wind was kicking up against us. Our heads were down going into the cold spray.

The subject matter is interesting, but the writing isn't. The passage is a series of short sentences, one after the other. When you have too many short sentences one after the other, try combining a few of them.

The result of combining some (but not all) short sentences is a paragraph whose sentences match the interest of the subject.

> On the first day Garth, Jim and I paddled fourteen kilometres down Johnstone Strait. We headed down the strait about five more kilometres to Robson Bight, a small bay well known for seeing dolphins. We paddled out into the strait so we could see the entire Bight, but there were no dolphins to be seen. By this time we were tired and hungry, the clouds had assumed a wintry dark thickness, and the wind was kicking up against us—our heads dropped going into the cold spray.

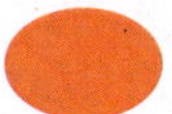

Eliminate Unnecessary Words

Clutter creeps into our lives every day. Clutter also creeps into writing through unnecessary words, inflated constructions and excessive jargon.

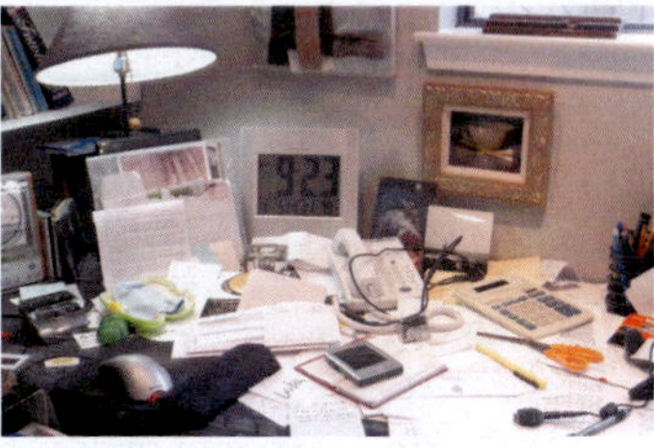

> **In regards to** the website, the content is **pretty** successful in **consideration of** the topic. The site is **fairly** good **writing-wise** and is **very** unique in telling you how to adjust the rear derailleur one step at a time.

The words in **red** are clutter. Get rid of the clutter. You can say the same thing with half the words and gain more impact as a result.

> The well-written website on bicycle repair provides step-by-step instructions on adjusting your rear derailleur.

Redundancy

Some words act as modifiers, but when you look closely at them they repeat the meaning of the word they pretend to modify. Have you heard someone refer to a *personal friend*? Aren't all friends personal? Likewise, you may have heard expressions such as *red in colour*, *small in size*, *round in shape* or *honest truth*. Imagine *red* not referring to colour or *round* not referring to shape.

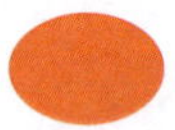

Reduce Wordy Phrases

Many inexperienced writers use phrases like 'It is my opinion that' or 'I think that' to begin sentences. These phrases are deadly to read. If you find them in your prose, cut them. Unless a writer is citing a source, we assume that the ideas are the writer's.

Coaches are among the worst at using many words for what could be said in a few:

> After much deliberation about Brown's future in rugby with regard to possible permanent injuries, I came to the conclusion that it would be in his best interest not to continue his pursuit of playing rugby again.

The coach might have said simply:

> Because Brown risks permanent injury if he plays rugby again, I decided to release him from the team.

Perhaps the coach wanted to sound impressive, authoritative or thoughtful. But the result is the opposite. Speakers and writers who impress us are those who use words efficiently.

COMMON ERRORS

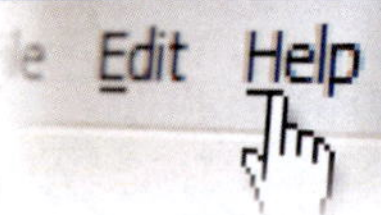

Empty intensifiers

Intensifiers modify verbs, adjectives and other adverbs, and they are often overused. One of the most overused intensifiers is *very.* Take the following sentence as an example:

> Her clothing style was **very unique**.

If something is unique, it is one of a kind. The word *very* doesn't make something more than unique.

> Her clothing style was **unique**.

or

> Her clothing style was **strange**.

COMMON ERRORS

Very and *totally* are but two of a list of empty intensifiers that can usually be eliminated with no loss of meaning. Other empty intensifiers include *absolutely*, *awfully*, *definitely*, *incredibly*, *particularly* and *really*.

Remember: When you use *very*, *totally* or another intensifier before an adjective or adverb, always ask yourself whether there is a more accurate adjective or adverb you could use instead to express the same thought.

WORDY PHRASES

Certain stock phrases plague writing in the workplace, in the media and in academia. Many can be replaced by one or two words with no loss in meaning.

Wordy	**Concise**
at this point in time	now
due to the fact that	because
for the purpose of	for
have the ability to	can
in order to	to
in spite of the fact that	although
in the event that	if

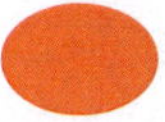

Simplify Tangled Sentences

Long sentences can be graceful and forceful. Such sentences, however, often require several revisions before they achieve elegance. Too often, long sentences reflect wandering thoughts that the writer didn't bother to go back and sort out. Two of the most important strategies for untangling long sentences are described in Chapter 18: Using active verbs (Section 18b) and Naming your agents (Section 18C). Here are some other strategies.

Revise expletives

Expletives are empty words that can occupy the subject position in a sentence. The most frequently used expletives are *there is*, *there are* and *it is*.

Wordy **There were** several important differences between the positions raised by the candidates in the debate.

To simplify the sentence, find the agent and make it the subject.

Revised The two **candidates** raised several important differences between their positions in the debate.

A few kinds of sentences—for example, *It is raining*—do require you to use an expletive. In most cases, however, expletives add unnecessary words, and sentences will read better without them.

Use positive constructions

Sentences become wordy and hard to read when they include two or more negatives such as the words *no*, *not* and *nor*, and the prefixes *un-* and *mis-*. For example:

Difficult A **not un**common complaint among employers of new university graduates is that they cannot communicate effectively in writing.

Revised Employers frequently complain that new university graduates cannot write effectively.

Even simpler Employers value the rare university graduate who can write well.

Phrasing sentences positively usually makes them more economical. Moreover, it makes your style more forceful and direct.

Simplify sentence structure

Long sentences can be hard to read, not because they are long but because they are convoluted and hide the relationships between ideas. Take the following sentence as an example.

> When the cessation of eight years of hostility in the Iran–Iraq war occurred in 1988, it was not the result of one side's defeating the other but the exhaustion of both after losing thousands of people and much of their military capability.

This sentence is hard to read. To rewrite sentences like this one, find the main ideas, then determine the relationships between them.

After examining the sentence, you decide there are two key ideas:

1. Iran and Iraq stopped fighting in 1988 after eight years.
2. Both sides were exhausted from losing people and equipment.

Next ask what the relationship is between the two ideas. When you identify the key ideas, the relationship is often obvious; in this case (2) is the cause of (1). Thus the word you want to connect the two ideas is *because.*

Iran and Iraq stopped fighting after eight years of an indecisive war **because** both sides had lost thousands of people and most of their equipment.

The revised sentence is both clearer and more concise, reducing the number of words from forty-two to twenty-five.

Photographs and writing gain energy when key ideas are emphasised.

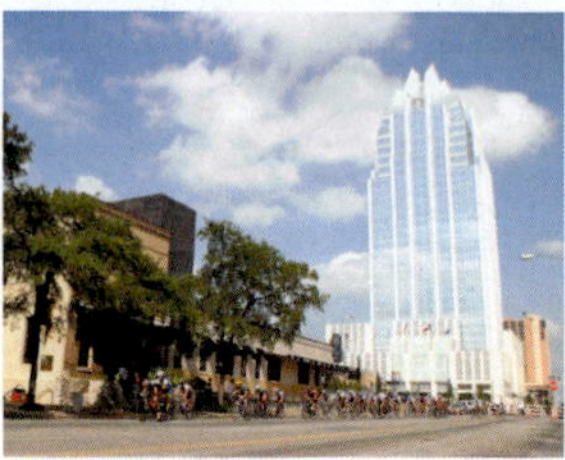

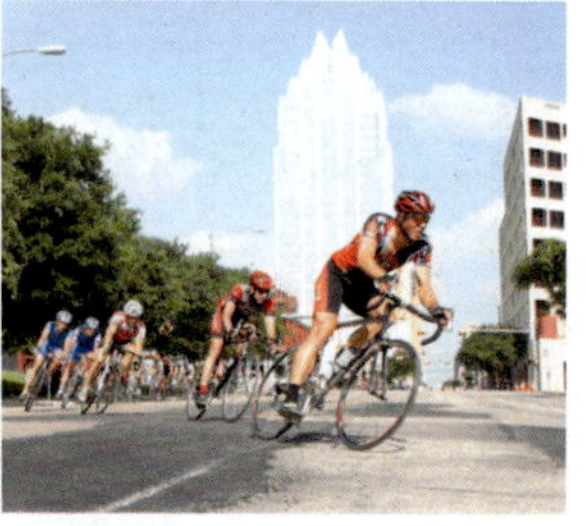

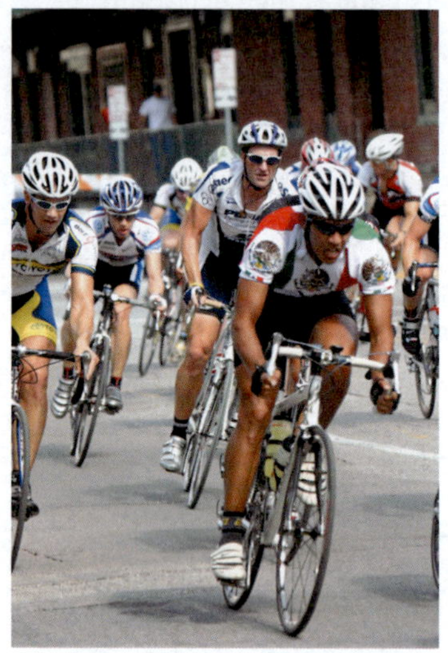

In visuals

Photographers create emphasis by composing the image to direct the attention of the viewer. Putting people and objects in the foreground and making them stand out against the background gives them emphasis.

In writing

Writers have many tools for creating emphasis. Writers can design a page to gain emphasis by using headings, white space, type size, colour and boldfacing. Just as important, learning the craft of structuring sentences will empower you to give your writing emphasis.

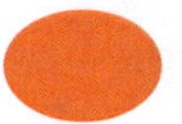

Manage Emphasis within Sentences

Put your main ideas in main clauses

Placing more important information in **main clauses** and less important information in subordinate clauses emphasises what is important.

In the following paragraph all the sentences are main clauses:

> Lotteries have been used to raise money for hundreds of years. Some lotteries ran into trouble. They were run by private companies. Sometimes the companies took off with the money. They didn't pay the winners.

This paragraph is grammatically correct, but it doesn't help the reader understand which pieces of information the author wants to emphasise. Combining the simple sentences into main and subordinate clauses and phrases can significantly improve the paragraph.

First, identify the main ideas:

> Lotteries have been used to raise money for hundreds of years.
> Some lotteries ran into trouble.

These ideas can be combined into one sentence:

> Lotteries have been used to raise money for hundreds of years, but some ran into trouble.

Now think about the relationship of the three remaining sentences to the main ideas. Those sentences explain why lotteries ran into trouble; thus the relationship is *because*.

> Lotteries have been used to raise money for hundreds of years, but some ran into trouble **because** they were run by private companies that sometimes took off with the money instead of paying the winners.

Put key ideas at the beginning and end of sentences

Read these sentences aloud:

1 The **Cottingley Fairies**, a series of five photographs taken in 1917 by Elsie Wright and Frances Griffiths, depicts the girls interacting with what seem to be fairies.

2 A series of photographs showing two girls interacting with what seem to be fairies, known as the **Cottingley Fairies**, was taken by Elsie Wright and Frances Griffiths in 1917.

3 The series of photos Elsie Wright and Frances Griffiths took in 1917 showing them interacting with what seem to be fairies is called the **Cottingley Fairies**.

Most readers put the primary emphasis on words at the beginning and end of a sentence. The front of a sentence usually gives what is known: the topic. At the back is the new information about the topic. Subordinate information is in the middle. If a paragraph is about the Cottingley Fairies, we would not expect the writer to choose sentence 2 over sentence 1 or 3. In sentence 2, the reference to the Cottingley Fairies is buried in the middle.

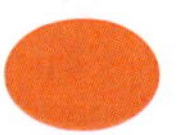

Forge Links across Sentences

When your writing maintains a focus of attention across sentences, the reader can distinguish the important ideas and how they relate to each other. To achieve this coherence, you need to control which ideas occupy the positions of greatest emphasis. The words you repeat from sentence to sentence act as links.

Link sentences from front to front

In front-to-front linkage, the subject of the sentence remains the focus from one sentence to the next. In the following sequence, sentences 1 to 5 are all about Arthur Wright. The subject of each sentence refers to the first sentence with the pronouns *he* and *his*.

1 **Arthur Wright** was one of the first electrical engineers in England.

2 **He** loaned his camera to his daughter Elsie, who took the fairy pictures in the yard behind their house.

3 **His** opinion was that the pictures were fake.

4 However, **his** wife, Polly, was convinced that they were real.

5 Nevertheless, **he** banned Elsie from ever using his camera again.

Each sentence adds more information about the repeated topic, Arthur Wright.

Link sentences from back to front

In back-to-front linkage, the new information at the end of the sentence is used as the topic of the next sentence. Back-to-front linkage allows new material to be introduced and commented on.

1 By summer of 1919, the girls and their photographs had become so well known that author Sir Arthur Conan Doyle even wrote an article for a leading magazine claiming that the photos and the fairies were **real**.

2 Not everyone believed that the Cottingley Fairies were **authentic**, however, and other public figures wrote to the papers calling the photographs a **hoax**.

3 The **hoax** continued until the 1980s, when both Elsie and Frances finally admitted that all but one of the pictures were fake.

Back-to-front linkage is useful when ideas need to be advanced quickly, as when you are telling stories. Rarely, however, will you use either front-to-front linkage or back-to-front linkage continuously throughout a piece of writing. Use front-to-front linkage to add more information and back-to-front linkage to move the topic along.

Check the links between your sentences to find any gaps that will cause your readers to stumble.

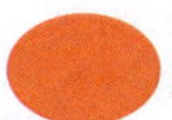

Use Parallel Structure with Parallel Ideas

What if Patrick Henry had written 'Give me liberty or I prefer not to live'? Would we remember those words today? We remember the words he did use: 'Give me liberty or give me death.' Writers who use parallel structure often create memorable sentences.

Use parallelism with *and*, *or*, *nor*, *but*

When you join elements at the same level with coordinating conjunctions, including *and*, *or*, *nor*, *yet*, *so*, *but* and *for*, normally you should use parallel grammatical structure for these elements.

Awkward

In today's global economy, **the method of production and where factories are located** has become relatively unimportant in comparison with **the creation of new concepts and marketing those concepts**.

Parallel

In today's global economy, **how goods are made and where they are produced** has become relatively unimportant in comparison with **creating new concepts and marketing those concepts**.

Use parallelism with *either/or, not only/but*

Make identical in structure the parts of sentences linked by correlative conjunctions: *either … or*, *neither … nor*, *not only … but also*, *whether … or*.

Awkward

Purchasing the undeveloped land not only **gives us a new park** but also it **is something that our children will benefit from in the future**.

Parallel

Purchasing the undeveloped land **will** not only **give our city a new park** but will **also leave our children a lasting inheritance**.

The more structural elements you match, the stronger the effect that parallelism will achieve.

COMMON ERRORS

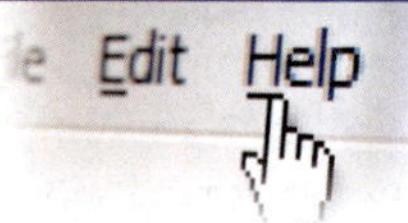

Faulty parallel structure

When writers neglect to use parallel structure, the result can be jarring. Reading your writing aloud will help you catch problems in parallelism. Read this sentence aloud:

At our club meeting we identified problems in **finding** new members, **publicising** our activities and **maintenance** of our website.

The end of the sentence doesn't sound right because the parallel structure is broken. We expect to find another verb + *ing* following *finding* and *publicising*. Instead, we run into *maintenance*, a noun. The problem is easy to fix: change the noun to the *-ing* verb form.

At our club meeting we identified problems in finding new members, publicising our activities and **maintaining** our website.

Remember: Use parallel structure for parallel ideas.

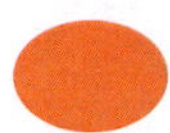

Be Aware of Levels of Formality

While you may get plenty of practice in informal writing—emails and notes to friends and family members—mastering formal writing is essential in academic and professional settings. How formal or informal should your writing be? That depends on your audience and the writing task at hand.

DECIDE HOW FORMAL YOUR WRITING SHOULD BE

- Who is your audience?
- What is the occasion?
- What level of formality is your audience accustomed to in similar situations?
- What impression of yourself do you want to give?

Colloquialisms

Colloquialisms are words or expressions that are used informally, often in conversation but less often in writing.

> I'm not happy with my essay mark, but that's the way **the cookie crumbles**.
>
> Liz is always **running off at the mouth** about something.
>
> I enjoyed the restaurant, but it was **nothing to write home about**.

In academic and professional writing, colloquialisms often suggest a flippant attitude, carelessness or even thoughtlessness. Sometimes colloquialisms can be used for ironic or humorous effect, but as a general rule, if you want to be taken seriously, avoid using them.

Avoiding colloquialisms doesn't mean, however, that you should use big words when small ones will do as well, or that you should use ten words instead of two. Formality doesn't mean being pretentious or wordy.

You can access the LTU information for academic writing here:
http://resource.unisa.edu.au/course/view.php?id=3633&topic=7

24 Final year of your program

By this stage of your studies you will have been exposed to different styles and approaches to academic writing.

Write an Observation

Observations are common in the natural sciences and in social science disciplines such as psychology, sociology and education. They begin as notes taken first-hand by the writer. Observations should include as many relevant and specific details as possible.

Elements of an observation

Title	Include a precise title.
Description and context	Be specific about what or whom you are observing. How did you limit your site or subject? What background information do readers need?
Record of observations	Report what you observed in some logical order: chronologically, from most obvious features to least obvious, or in some other pattern.
Conclusion or summary	Give your readers a framework in which to understand your observations. What conclusions can you draw from them? What questions are left unanswered?

What you need to do

- Carry a notebook and make extensive field notes. Provide as much information as possible about the activities you observe.
- Record in your notebook or mobile device if you prefer exactly when you arrived and left, where you were, and exactly what you saw and heard.
- Analyse your observations before you write about them. Identify patterns, and organise your report according to those patterns. Situate your analysis in the literature of the discipline.

25 Writing for nursing practice

Writing for nursing practice is very different from academic writing, but the principles of good writing are the same. It is a form of communication and you have to be very aware of your reader audience.

Writing for nursing practice involves writing reports describing a patient's clinical condition/state of health. You will be writing for a multidisciplinary team, so your report must be clear, concise and able to be understood by all health professionals. Below are some guidelines for effective nursing documentation:

- All entries should be accurate and factual
- Make corrections as required under hospital policies – information should not be deleted – with electronic documentation this would be easy to do
- All information should be timely and relevant
- All nursing interventions and the interventions of other health professionals have to be evaluated and this documented
- All patient health care and social issues (if relevant) must be documented
- All charting must be objective. Document within specific clinical and/or psycho-social parameters
- All nursing noted need to be legible (if handwritten) and reflect the patient's clinical condition.

26 Presenting your work

Throughout your undergraduate program you will be required to present aspects of your work to fellow students and to your lecturer(s). This is usually an assessment item for one of your courses. Most people have a fear of public speaking, including students, but this is a part of preparing you for professional practice.

The key to successful oral presentations is preparedness. You prepare for your oral presentation in much the same way as you do for a written assignment.

- You research the topic
- Identify key points/ideas
- Prepare your Power Point slides; YouTube; film etc. and

then you practice presenting the information. The more you practice the less nervous you will be.

You already know your audience: fellow students and your lecturer. In some courses the oral presentations are peer assessed which means that your fellow students will be assessing your presentation according to marking criteria. These criteria will include:

- **Structure of the presentation:** introduction, content, summary. So it is important to grab the attention of the audience from the beginning. The content should be relevant to the topic and the summary should be a restatement of main points.
- **Delivery of the material**: the use of teaching aids; props if appropriate. Remember props should not detract from your presentation.
- **Voice:** your voice must reach the people in the back row of the lecture venue so knowing how to the microphone is something you will have to learn if you do not know how. Do not mumble, speak clearly, make eye contact with everyone in the audience- DO NOT FOCUS on one person or spot.

As a part of your preparation watch stand- up comedians as they perform in front of a live audience: how they engage the audience; how they project their voice but most importantly how they time their delivery. Timing your delivery is very important because you have to allow time for your audience to take in the information; understand it and make sense of it. So if you deliver all of your material in less than a minute it may influence your grade.

Always allow time for questions from the audience- 2-3 minutes at most for a student presentation. So if you have been allocated 10 minutes for your presentation then your presentation will take 7-8 minutes allowing time for questions. So you can see the importance of timing in oral presentations. It is not a good practice to go over time because audiences get bored and it disadvantages the next speaker.

Always ask for feedback- if this oral presentation is an assessment item then there should be a feedback sheet provided that your class may have helped develop.

27 Poster presentations

These may be an assessment item for some courses including research courses. The poster is a visual representation of key ideas/points around a specific topic. Posters provide an overview of a topic. Posters "are a recognised form of knowledge transfer" (Rowe, Ilic 2011, p. 210). For those of you who have been to conferences you will have seen posters presented that reflect the conference themes. Your school/faculty will also have posters on walls of work completed by other students and lecturers. Below are two examples of research posters.

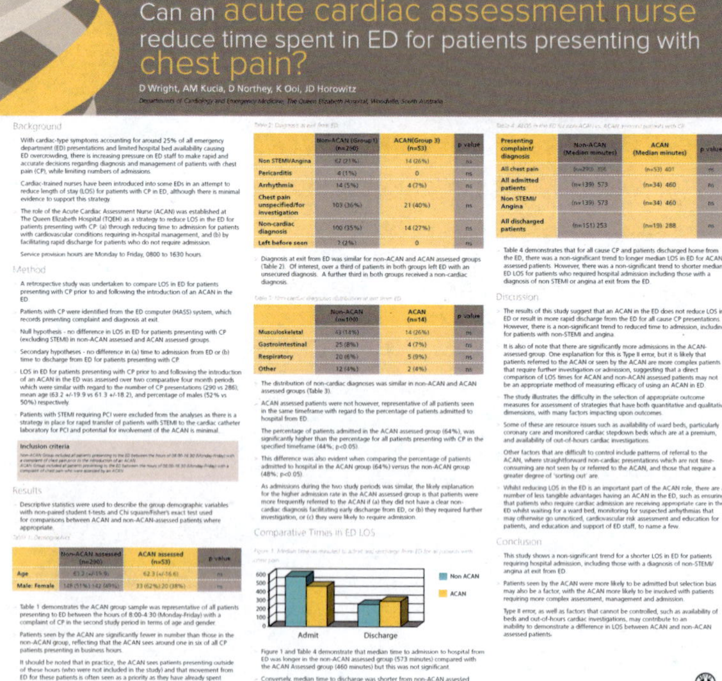

Can an acute cardiac assessment nurse reduce time spent in ED for patients presenting with chest pain?

D Wright, AM Kucia, D Northey, K Ooi, JD Horowitz

Departments of Cardiology and Emergency Medicine, The Queen Elizabeth Hospital, Woodville, South Australia

Background

- With cardiac-type symptoms accounting for around 25% of all emergency department (ED) presentations and limited hospital bed availability causing ED overcrowding, there is increasing pressure on ED staff to make rapid and accurate decisions regarding diagnosis and management of patients with chest pain (CP), while limiting numbers of admissions.
- Cardiac-trained nurses have been introduced into some EDs in an attempt to reduce length of stay (LOS) for patients with CP in ED, although there is minimal evidence to support this strategy.
- The role of the Acute Cardiac Assessment Nurse (ACAN) was established at The Queen Elizabeth Hospital (TQEH) as a strategy to reduce LOS in the ED for patients presenting with CP: (a) through reducing time to admission for patients with cardiovascular conditions requiring in-hospital management, and (b) by facilitating rapid discharge for patients who do not require admission.
- Service provision hours are Monday to Friday, 0800 to 1630 hours.

Method

- A retrospective study was undertaken to compare LOS in ED for patients presenting with CP prior to and following the introduction of an ACAN in the ED.
- Patients with CP were identified from the ED computer (HASS) system, which records presenting complaint and diagnosis at exit.
- Null hypothesis - no difference in LOS in ED for patients presenting with CP (excluding STEMI) in non-ACAN assessed and ACAN assessed groups.
- Secondary hypotheses - no difference in (a) time to admission from ED or (b) time to discharge from ED for patients presenting with CP.
- LOS in ED for patients presenting with CP prior to and following the introduction of an ACAN in the ED was assessed over two comparative four month periods which were similar with regard to the number of CP presentations (290 vs 286), mean age (63.2 +/-19.9 vs 61.3 +/-18.2), and percentage of males (52% vs 50%) respectively.
- Patients with STEMI requiring PCI were excluded from the analyses as there is a strategy in place for rapid transfer of patients with STEMI to the cardiac catheter laboratory for PCI and potential for involvement of the ACAN is minimal.

Inclusion criteria

Non-ACAN Group included all patients presenting to the ED between the hours of 08:00-16:30 (Monday-Friday) with a complaint of chest pain prior to the introduction of an ACAN.
ACAN Group included all patients presenting to the ED between the hours of 08:00-16:30 (Monday-Friday) with a complaint of chest pain who were assessed by an ACAN.

Results

- Descriptive statistics were used to describe the group demographic variables with non-paired student t-tests and Chi square/Fisher's exact test used for comparisons between ACAN and non-ACAN-assessed patients where appropriate.

Table 1: Demographics

	Non-ACAN assessed (n=290)	ACAN assessed (n=53)	p value
Age	63.2 (+/-19.9)	62.3 (+/-16.6)	ns
Male: Female	148 (51%):142 (49%)	33 (62%):20 (38%)	ns

- Table 1 demonstrates the ACAN group sample was representative of all patients presenting to ED between the hours of 8:00-4:30 (Monday-Friday) with a complaint of CP in the second study period in terms of age and gender.
- Patients seen by the ACAN are significantly fewer in number than those in the non-ACAN group, reflecting that the ACAN sees around one in six of all CP patients presenting in business hours.
- It should be noted that in practice, the ACAN sees patients presenting outside of these hours (who were not included in the study) and that movement from ED for these patients is often seen as a priority as they have already spent several hours in the ED. The ACAN also sees patients with other cardiovascular complaints, such as those with heart failure or collapse thought to be due to arrhythmia.

Table 2: Diagnosis at exit from ED

	Non-ACAN (Group1) (n=290)	ACAN(Group 3) (n=53)	p value
Non STEMI/Angina	67 (21%)	14 (26%)	ns
Pericarditis	4 (1%)	0	ns
Arrhythmia	14 (5%)	4 (7%)	ns
Chest pain unspecified/for investigation	103 (36%)	21 (40%)	ns
Non-cardiac diagnosis	100 (35%)	14 (27%)	ns
Left before seen	7 (2%)	0	ns

- Diagnosis at exit from ED was similar for non-ACAN and ACAN assessed groups (Table 2). Of interest, over a third of patients in both groups left ED with an unsecured diagnosis. A further third in both groups received a non-cardiac diagnosis.

Table 3: Non-cardiac diagnoses distribution at exit from ED

	Non-ACAN (n=100)	ACAN (n=14)	p value
Musculoskeletal	43 (14%)	14 (26%)	ns
Gastrointestinal	25 (8%)	4 (7%)	ns
Respiratory	20 (6%)	5 (9%)	ns
Other	12 (4%)	2 (4%)	ns

- The distribution of non-cardiac diagnoses was similar in non-ACAN and ACAN assessed groups (Table 3).
- ACAN assessed patients were not however, representative of all patients seen in the same timeframe with regard to the percentage of patients admitted to hospital from ED.
- The percentage of patients admitted in the ACAN assessed group (64%), was significantly higher than the percentage for all patients presenting with CP in the specified timeframe (44%; p<0.05).
- This difference was also evident when comparing the percentage of patients admitted to hospital in the ACAN group (64%) versus the non-ACAN group (48%; p<0.05).
- As admissions during the two study periods was similar, the likely explanation for the higher admission rate in the ACAN assessed group is that patients were more frequently referred to the ACAN if (a) they did not have a clear non-cardiac diagnosis facilitating early discharge from ED, or (b) they required further investigation, or (c) they were likely to require admission.

Comparative Times in ED LOS

Figure 1: Median time (in minutes) to admit and discharge from ED for all patients with chest pain

- Figure 1 and Table 4 demonstrate that median time to admission to hospital from ED was longer in the non-ACAN assessed group (573 minutes) compared with the ACAN Assessed group (460 minutes) but this was not significant.
- Conversely, median time to discharge was shorter from non-ACAN assessed patients (253 minutes) compared with the ACAN assessed group (288 minutes). Again this was not significant.

Table 4: ALOS in the ED for non-ACAN vs. ACAN assessed patients with CP

Presenting complaint/ diagnosis	Non-ACAN (Median minutes)	ACAN (Median minutes)	p value
All chest pain	(n=290) 356	(n=53) 401	ns
All admitted patients	(n=139) 573	(n=34) 460	ns
Non STEMI/ Angina	(n=139) 573	(n=34) 460	ns
All discharged patients	(n=151) 253	(n=19) 288	ns

- Table 4 demonstrates that for all cause CP and patients discharged home from the ED, there was a non-significant trend to longer median LOS in ED for ACAN-assessed patients. However, there was a non-significant trend to shorter median ED LOS for patients who required hospital admission including those with a diagnosis of non STEMI or angina at exit from the ED.

Discussion

- The results of this study suggest that an ACAN in the ED does not reduce LOS in ED or result in more rapid discharge from the ED for all cause CP presentations. However, there is a non-significant trend to reduced time to admission, including for patients with non-STEMI and angina.
- It is also of note that there are significantly more admissions in the ACAN-assessed group. One explanation for this is Type II error, but it is likely that patients referred to the ACAN or seen by the ACAN are more complex patients that require further investigation or admission, suggesting that a direct comparison of LOS times for ACAN and non-ACAN assessed patients may not be an appropriate method of measuring efficacy of using an ACAN in ED.
- The study illustrates the difficulty in the selection of appropriate outcome measures for assessment of strategies that have both quantitative and qualitative dimensions, with many factors impacting upon outcomes.
- Some of these are resource issues such as availability of ward beds, particularly coronary care and monitored cardiac stepdown beds which are at a premium, and availability of out-of-hours cardiac investigations.
- Other factors that are difficult to control include patterns of referral to the ACAN, where straightforward non-cardiac presentations which are not time-consuming are not seen by or referred to the ACAN, and those that require a greater degree of 'sorting out' are.
- Whilst reducing LOS in the ED is an important part of the ACAN role, there are a number of less tangible advantages having an ACAN in the ED, such as ensuring that patients who require cardiac admission are receiving appropriate care in the ED whilst waiting for a ward bed, monitoring for suspected arrhythmias that may otherwise go unnoticed, cardiovascular risk assessment and education for patients, and education and support of ED staff, to name a few.

Conclusion

- This study shows a non-significant trend for a shorter LOS in ED for patients requiring hospital admission, including those with a diagnosis of non-STEMI/angina at exit from ED.
- Patients seen by the ACAN were more likely to be admitted but selection bias may also be a factor, with the ACAN more likely to be involved with patients requiring more complex assessment, management and admission.
- Type II error, as well as factors that cannot be controlled, such as availability of beds and out-of-hours cardiac investigations, may contribute to an inability to demonstrate a difference in LOS between ACAN and non-ACAN assessed patients.

Government of South Australia
SA Health

Tips for developing a Poster Presentation

- Posters are just as important as presenting papers so ensure your poster information is rigorous and robust
- Posters need to attract your audience- people will look at posters that grab their interest
- Your poster presents your ideas and work to others so make it interesting
- Do not overfill your poster with text- the poster information is concise and to the point
- Be familiar with your topic- you may have to present the poster information in less than a minute
- Provide hyperlinks to supporting information
- Your poster should be aesthetically pleasing
- Information to include on your poster:
- Title
- Background
- Overview
- Key points
- Summary
- Conclusion
- References
- Your contact details

References

Allen, M 2012, *Smart Thinking*, Oxford University Press, Australia.

Crisp, GT. 2012. *Integrative Assessment: reframing assessment practice for current and future learning. Assessment & Evaluation in Higher education*, 37:1, 33-43.

Faigley, L 2013, *The Little Penguin Handbook*. 2nd edition, Pearson Australia , Sydney.

Ragusa, A 2012, *Writing for the social sciences*. Pearson Australia, Sydney.

Rowe, N & Ilic, D 2011. *Poster presentation – a visual medium for academic and scientific meetings Paediatric Respiratory Reviews* 12 (2011), pp. 208–213.

Wright D, Kucia, AM, Northey D, Ooi K. Horowitz, JD 2009. Department of Cardiology & Emergency Medicine, The Queen Elizabeth Hospital Woodville South Australia.

Glossary of Grammatical Terms and Usage

The glossary gives the definitions of grammatical terms and items of usage. The grammatical terms are shown in **blue**. Some of the explanations of usage that follow are not rules but guidelines to keep in mind for academic and professional writing. In these formal contexts, the safest course is to avoid words that are described as *non-standard*, *informal* or *colloquial*.

a/an Use *a* before words that begin with a consonant sound (*a train*, *a house*). Use *an* before words that begin with a vowel sound (*an avocado*, *an hour*).

a lot/alot *A lot* is generally regarded as informal; *alot* is not a word.

accept/except *Accept* is a verb meaning 'receive' or 'approve'. *Except* is sometimes a verb meaning 'leave out', but much more often it is used as a conjunction or preposition meaning 'other than'.

active A clause with a transitive verb in which the subject is the doer of the action (see Section 18a). See also **passive**.

adjective A modifier that qualifies or describes the qualities of a noun or pronoun (see Sections 27a and 27b).

adjective clause A subordinate clause that modifies a noun or pronoun and is usually introduced by a relative pronoun (see Section 27b). Sometimes called a *relative clause*.

adverb A word that modifies a verb, another modifier or a clause (see Sections 27a and 27c).

adverb clause A subordinate clause that functions as an adverb by modifying a verb, another modifier or a clause (see Section 27c).

advice/advise The noun *advice* means a 'suggestion'; the verb *advise* means to 'recommend' or 'give advice'.

affect/effect Usually, *affect* is a verb (to 'influence') and *effect* is a noun (a 'result'). Less commonly, *affect* is used as a noun and *effect* as a verb.

agreement The number and person of a subject and verb must match—singular subjects with singular verbs, plural subjects with plural verbs (see Chapter 23). Likewise, the number and gender of a pronoun and its antecedent must match (see Section 25b).

all ready/already The adjective phrase *all ready* means 'completely prepared'; the adverb *already* means 'previously'.

all right/alright *All right*, meaning 'acceptable', is the correct spelling. *Alright* is non-standard.

allude/elude *Allude* means 'refer to indirectly'. *Elude* means 'evade'.

allusion/illusion An *allusion* is an indirect reference; an *illusion* is a false impression.

among/between *Between* refers to precisely two people or things; *among* refers to three or more.

amount/number Use *amount* with things that cannot be counted; use *number* with things that can be counted.

an See **a/an**.

antecedent The noun (or pronoun) that a pronoun refers to (see Section 25b).

anybody/any body; anyone/any one *Anybody* and *anyone* are indefinite pronouns and have the same meaning. In *any body*, *body* is a noun modified by *any*, and in *any one*, *one* is a pronoun or adjective modified by *any*.

anymore/any more *Anymore* means 'now', while *any more* means 'no more'. Both are used in negative constructions.

anyway/anyways *Anyway* is correct. *Anyways* is non-standard.

articles The words *a*, *an* and *the* (see Section 28b).

as/as if/as though/like Use *as* instead of *like* before dependent clauses (which include a subject and verb). Use *like* before a noun or a pronoun.

assure/ensure/insure *Assure* means 'promise', *ensure* means 'make certain', and *insure* means to 'make certain in either a legal or a financial sense'.

auxiliary verb Forms of *be*, *do* and *have* combine with verbs to indicate tense and mood (see Section 28c). The modal verbs *can*, *could*, *may*, *might*, *must*, *shall*, *should*, *will* and *would* are a subset of auxiliaries.

bad/badly Use *bad* only as an adjective. *Badly* is the adverb.

being as/being that Both constructions are colloquial and awkward substitutes for *because*. Don't use them in formal writing.

beside/besides *Beside* means 'next to'. *Besides* means 'in addition to' or 'except'.

between See **among/between**.

bring/take *Bring* describes movement from a more distant location to a nearer one. *Take* describes movement away.

can/may In formal writing, *can* indicates ability or capacity, while *may* indicates permission.

case The form of a noun or pronoun that indicates its function. Nouns change case only to show possession: the dog, the dog's bowl. See **pronoun case** (Section 25a).

censor/censure To *censor* is to edit or ban on moral or political grounds. To *censure* is to reprimand publicly.

cite/sight/site To *cite* is to 'mention specifically'; *sight* as a verb means to 'observe' and as a noun refers to 'vision'; *site* is most commonly used as a noun that means 'location', but it is also used as a verb to mean 'situate'.

clause A group of words with a subject and a predicate. A main or independent clause can stand as a sentence. A subordinate or dependent clause must be attached to a main clause to form a sentence (see Section 22a).

collective noun A noun that refers to a group or a plurality, such as *team*, *army* or *committee* (see Section 23d).

comma splice Two independent clauses joined incorrectly by a comma (see Section 22c).

common noun A noun that names a general group, person, place or thing (see Section 28a). Common nouns are not capitalised unless they begin a sentence.

complement A word or group of words that completes the predicate. See also **linking verb**.

complement/compliment To *complement* something is to complete it or make it perfect; to *compliment* is to flatter.

complex sentence A sentence that contains at least one subordinate clause attached to a main clause.

compound sentence A sentence that contains at least two main clauses.

compound-complex sentence A sentence that contains at least two main clauses and one subordinate clause.

conjunction See **coordinating conjunction** and **subordinating conjunction**.

conjunctive adverb An adverb that often modifies entire clauses and sentences, such as *also*, *consequently*, *however*, *indeed*, *instead*, *moreover*, *nevertheless*, *otherwise*, *similarly* and *therefore* (see Section 27c).

continual/continuous *Continual* refers to a repeated activity; *continuous* refers to an ongoing, unceasing activity.

coordinate A relationship of equal importance, in terms of either grammar or meaning (see Section 20c).

coordinating conjunction A word that links two equivalent grammatical elements, such as *and*, *but*, *or*, *yet*, *nor*, *for* and *so*.

could of Non-standard. See **have/of**.

countable noun A noun that names things that can be counted, such as *block*, *cat* and *toy* (see Section 28a).

dangling modifier A modifier that isn't clearly attached to what it modifies (see Section 27e).

data The plural form of *datum*; it takes plural verb forms.

declarative A sentence that makes a statement.

dependent clause See **subordinate clause**.

determiners Words that initiate noun phrases, including possessive nouns (*Paul's*); possessive pronouns (*my*, *your*); demonstrative pronouns (*this*, *that*); and indefinite pronouns (*all, both, many*).

differ from/differ with To *differ from* means to 'be unlike'; to *differ with* means to 'disagree'.

different from/different than Use *different from* where possible.

Dark French roast is **different from** ordinary coffee.

direct object A noun, pronoun or noun clause that names who or what receives the action of a transitive verb.

discreet/discrete Both are adjectives. *Discreet* means 'prudent' or 'tactful'; *discrete* means 'separate'.

disinterested/uninterested *Disinterested* is often misused to mean *uninterested.* Disinterested means 'impartial'. A judge can be interested in a case but disinterested in the outcome.

double negative The incorrect use of two negatives to signal the same negative meaning.

due to the fact that Avoid this wordy substitute for *because*.

each other/one another Use *each other* for two; use *one another* for more than two.

effect See **affect/effect**.

elicit/illicit The verb *elicit* means to 'draw out'. The adjective *illicit* means 'unlawful'.

emigrate from/immigrate to *Emigrate* means to 'leave one's country'; *immigrate* means to 'settle in another country'.

ensure See **assure/ensure/insure**.

enthused Non-standard in academic and professional writing. Use *enthusiastic* instead.

etc. Avoid this abbreviation for the Latin *et cetera* in formal writing. Either list all the items or use an English phrase such as *and so forth*.

every body/everybody; every one/everyone *Everybody* and *everyone* are indefinite pronouns referring to all people under discussion. *Every one* and *every body* are adjective–noun combinations referring to all members of a group.

except See **accept/except**.

except for the fact that Avoid this wordy substitute for *except that*.

expletive The dummy subjects *it* and *there* used to fill a grammatical slot in a sentence. ***It*** *is raining outside.* ***There*** *should be a law against it.*

explicit/implicit Both are adjectives; *explicit* means 'stated outright', while *implicit* means just the opposite, 'unstated'.

farther/further *Farther* refers to physical distance; *further* refers to time or other abstract concepts.

fewer/less Use *fewer* with what can be counted and *less* with what cannot be counted.

flunk In formal writing, avoid this colloquial substitute for *fail*.

fragment A group of words beginning with a capital letter and ending with a full stop that looks like a sentence but lacks a subject or a predicate or both (see Section 22a).

further See **farther/further**.

gerund An *-ing* form of a verb used as a noun, such as *running*, *skiing* or *laughing*.

good/well *Good* is an adjective and is not interchangeable with the adverb *well*. The one exception is health. Both she feels *good* and she feels *well* are correct.

hanged/hung Use *hanged* to refer only to executions; *hung* is used for all other instances.

have/of *Have*, not *of*, follows *should*, *could*, *would*, *may*, *must* and *might*.

he/she; s/he Try to avoid language that appears to exclude either gender (unless this is intended, of course) and awkward compromises such as *he/she* or *s/he*. The best solution is to make pronouns plural (the gender-neutral *they*) wherever possible (see Section 25c).

helping verb See **auxiliary verb**.

hopefully This adverb is commonly used as a sentence modifier, but many readers object to it.

illusion See **allusion/illusion**.

immigrate See **emigrate from/immigrate to**.

imperative A sentence that expresses a command. Usually the subject is implied rather than stated.

implicit See **explicit/implicit**.

imply/infer *Imply* means to 'suggest'; *infer* means to 'draw a conclusion'.

in regards to Avoid this wordy substitute for *regarding*.

incredible/incredulous *Incredible* means 'unbelievable'; *incredulous* means 'not believing'.

independent clause See **main clause**.

indirect object A noun, pronoun or noun clause that names who or what is affected by the action of a transitive verb.

infinitive The word *to* plus the base verb form: *to believe, to feel, to act*. See also **split infinitive**.

infinitive phrase A phrase that uses the infinitive form of a verb.

interjection A word expressing feeling that is grammatically unconnected to a sentence, such as *cool, wow, ouch* or *yikes*.

interrogative A sentence that asks a question.

intransitive verb A verb that doesn't take an object, such as *sleep, appear* or *laugh* (see Sections 24c and 28c).

irregardless Non-standard for *regardless*.

irregular verb A verb that doesn't use either *-d* or *-ed* to form the past tense and past participle (see Section 24b).

-ise/-wise The suffix *-ise* changes a noun or adjective into a verb (*harmony, harmonise*). The suffix *-wise* changes a noun or adjective into an adverb (*clock, clockwise*). Some writers are tempted to use these suffixes to convert almost any word into an adverb or verb form. Unless the word appears in a dictionary, don't use it.

it is my opinion that Avoid this wordy substitute for *I believe that.*

its/it's *Its* is the possessive of *it* and doesn't take an apostrophe; *it's* is the contraction for *it is.*

kind of/sort of/type of Avoid using these colloquial expressions if you mean *somewhat* or *rather*. *It's kind of hot* is non-standard. Each is permissible, however, when it refers to a classification of an object. Be sure that it agrees in number with the object it is modifying.

lay/lie *Lay* means 'place' or 'put' and generally takes a direct object (see Section 24c). Its main forms are *lay, laid, laid. Lie* means 'recline' or 'be positioned' and doesn't take an object. Its main forms are *lie, lay, lain.*

less See **fewer**.

lie See **lay/lie**.

linking verb A verb that connects the subject to the complement, such as *appear, be, feel, look, seem* or *taste*.

lots/lots of Non-standard in formal writing; use *many* or *much* instead.

main clause A group of words with a subject and a predicate that can stand alone as a sentence. Also called an *independent clause.*

mankind This term offends some readers and is outdated. Use *humans, humanity* or *people* instead.

may/can See **can/may**.

may be/maybe *May be* is a verb phrase; *maybe* is an adverb.

media This is the plural form of the noun *medium* and requires a plural verb.

might of See **have/of**.

modal A kind of auxiliary verb that indicates ability, permission, intention, obligation or probability, such as *can*, *could*, *may*, *might*, *must*, *shall*, *should*, *will* or *would*.

modifier A general term for adjectives, adverbs, phrases and clauses that describe other words (see Chapter 27).

must of See **have/of**.

non-restrictive modifier A modifier that isn't essential to the meaning of the word, phrase or clause it modifies and should be set off by commas or other punctuation (see Section 29c).

noun The name of a person, place, thing, concept or action. See also **common noun** and **proper noun** (see Section 28a).

noun clause A subordinate clause that functions as a noun.

number See **amount/number**.

object Receiver of the action within the clause or phrase.

OK, okay Informal; avoid using in academic and professional writing. Each spelling is accepted in informal usage.

owing to the fact that Avoid this wordy, colloquial substitute for *because*.

parallelism The principle of putting similar elements or ideas in similar grammatical form (see Section 20c).

participle A form of a verb that uses *-ing* in the present (*laughing*, *playing*) and usually *-ed* or *-en* in the past (*laughed*, *played*). See Section 24a. Participles are either part of the verb phrase (*She had played the game before*) or used as adjectives (*the laughing girl*).

participial phrase A phrase formed either by a present participle (for example, *racing*) or by a past participle (for example, *taken*).

parts of speech The eight classes of words according to their grammatical function: nouns, pronouns, verbs, adjectives, adverbs, prepositions, conjunctions and interjections.

passive A clause with a transitive verb in which the subject is being acted upon (see Section 18a). See also **active**.

people/persons *People* refers to a general group; *persons* refers to a collection of individuals. Use *people* over *persons* except when you are emphasising the idea of separate persons within the group.

per Try not to use the English equivalent of this Latin word except in technical writing or familiar usages such as *kilometres per litre*.

phenomena This is the plural form of *phenomenon* ('observable fact' or 'unusual event') and takes plural verbs.

phrase A group of words that doesn't contain both a subject and a predicate.

plenty In academic and professional writing, avoid this colloquial substitute for *very*.

plus Don't use *plus* to join clauses or sentences. Use *and, also, moreover, furthermore* or another conjunctive adverb instead.

precede/proceed Both are verbs but they have different meanings: *precede* means 'come before', and *proceed* means 'go ahead' or 'continue'.

predicate The part of the clause that expresses the action or tells something about the subject. The predicate includes the verb and all its complements, objects and modifiers.

prejudice/prejudiced *Prejudice* is a noun; *prejudiced* is an adjective.

preposition A class of words that indicate relationships and qualities.

prepositional phrase A phrase formed by a preposition and its object, including the modifiers of its object.

pronoun A word that stands for other nouns or pronouns. Pronouns have several subclasses, including personal pronouns, possessive pronouns, demonstrative pronouns, indefinite pronouns, relative pronouns, interrogative pronouns, reflexive pronouns and reciprocal pronouns (Chapter 25).

pronoun case Pronouns that function as the subjects of sentences are in the subjective case (*I, you, he, she, it, we, they*). Pronouns that function as direct or indirect objects are in the objective case (*me, you, him, her, it, us, them*). Pronouns that indicate ownership are in the possessive case (*my, your, his, her, its, our, their*) (see Section 25a).

proper noun A noun that names a particular person, place, thing or group (see Section 28a). Proper nouns are capitalised.

question as to whether/question of whether Avoid these wordy substitutes for *whether*.

raise/rise The verb *raise* means 'lift up' and takes a direct object. Its main forms are *raise, raised, raised*. The verb *rise* means 'get up' and doesn't take a direct object. Its main forms are *rise, rose, risen*.

real/really Avoid using *real* as if it were an adverb. *Really* is an adverb; *real* is an adjective.

reason is because Omit either *reason is* or *because* when explaining causality.

reason why Avoid using this redundant combination.

relative pronoun A pronoun that initiates clauses, such as *that, which, what, who, whom* or *whose*.

restrictive modifier A modifier that is essential to the meaning of the word, phrase or clause it modifies (see Section 29c). Restrictive modifiers are usually not set off by punctuation.

rise/raise See **raise/rise**.

run-on sentence Two main clauses fused together without punctuation or a conjunction, appearing as one sentence (see Section 22b).

sentence A grammatically independent group of words that contains at least one main clause.

sentence fragment See **fragment**.

set/sit *Set* means 'put' and takes a direct object; its main forms are *set, set, set. Sit* means 'be seated' and doesn't take a direct object; its main forms are *sit, sat, sat. Sit* should not be used as a synonym for *set*.

shall/will *Shall* is used most often in first person questions, while *will* is a future tense helping verb for all persons. British English consistently uses *shall* with first person: *I shall, we shall*.

should of See **have/of**.

sit/set See **set/sit**.

some time/sometime/sometimes *Some time* means 'a span of time', *sometime* means 'at some unspecified time', and *sometimes* means 'occasionally'.

somebody/some body; someone/some one *Somebody* and *someone* are indefinite pronouns and have the same meaning. In *some body, body* is a noun modified by *some*, and in *some one, one* is a pronoun or adjective modified by *some*.

sort of See **kind of/sort of/type of**.

split infinitive An infinitive with a word or words between *to* and the base verb form, such as *to boldly go, to better appreciate*.

stationary/stationery *Stationary* means 'motionless'; *stationery* means 'writing paper'.

subject A noun, pronoun or noun phrase that identifies what the clause is about and connects with the predicate.

subject–verb agreement See **agreement**.

subordinate A relationship of unequal importance, in terms of either grammar or meaning (see Section 20a).

subordinate clause A clause that cannot stand alone but must be attached to a main clause. Also called a *dependent clause*.

subordinating conjunction A word that introduces a subordinate clause. Common subordinating conjunctions are *after, although, as, because, before, if, since, that, unless, until, when, where* and *while*.

such Avoid using *such* as a synonym for *very*. *Such* should always be followed by *that* and a clause that contains a result.

sure A colloquial term used as an adverb to mean 'certainly'. Avoid using it this way in formal writing.

sure and/sure to; try and/try to *Sure to* and *try to* are correct; don't use *and* after *sure* or *try*.

take See **bring/take**.

that/which *That* introduces a restrictive or essential clause. Restrictive clauses describe an object that must be that particular object and no other. Though some writers occasionally use *which* with restrictive clauses, it is most often used to introduce non-restrictive clauses. These are clauses that contain additional non-essential information about the object (see Section 29c).

transition A word or phrase that notes movement from one unit of writing to another.

transitive verb A verb that takes a direct object (see Section 24c).

uncountable noun A noun that names things that cannot be counted, such as *air*, *energy* or *water* (see Section 28a).

verb A word that expresses action or characterises the subject in some way. Verbs can show tense and mood (see Chapter 24 and Section 28c).

verbal A form of a verb used as an adjective, adverb or noun. See also **gerund**, **infinitive**, **participle**.

well/good See **good/well**.

which/that See **that/which**.

who/whom *Who* and *whom* follow the same rules as other pronouns: *Who* is the subject pronoun; *whom* is the object pronoun (see Section 25a).

will/shall See **shall/will**.

-wise/-ise See **-ise/-wise**.

would of See **have/of**.

you Avoid indefinite uses of *you*. It should only be used to mean 'you, the reader'.

your/you're The two are not interchangeable. *Your* is the possessive form of 'you'; *you're* is the contraction of 'you are'.